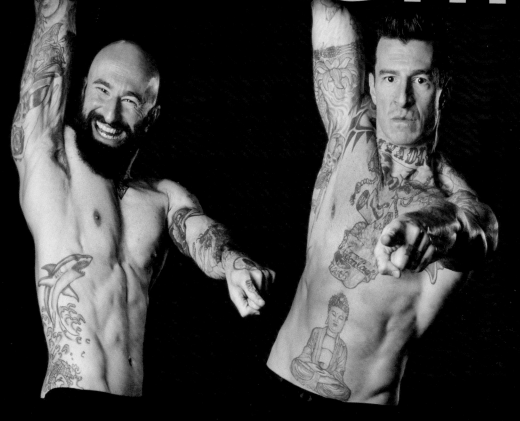

Next Le STRENGTH

The Ultimate Rings and Parallettes Program

AL KAVADLO & DANNY KAVADLO

Next Level STRENGTH

The Ultimate Rings and Parallettes Program

AL KAVADLO & DANNY KAVADLO

A Dragon Door Publications, Inc. production

All rights under International and Pan-American Copyright conventions.

Published in the United States by: Dragon Door Publications, Inc.

5 East County Rd B, #3 • Little Canada, MN 55117

Tel: (651) 487-2180 • Fax: (651) 487-3954

Credit card orders: 1-800-899-5111 • Email: support@dragondoor.com • Website: www.dragondoor.com

ISBN 10: 1-942812-17-5   ISBN 13: 978-1-942812-17-3

This edition first published in May 2019

Printed in China

BOOK DESIGN: Derek Brigham • www.dbrigham.com • bigd@dbrigham.com

PHOTOGRAPHY: M. Nuri Shakoor, Urban Art by Nuri Photography

ADDITIONAL PHOTOGRAPHY: Michael Alago, Tania Amador, Riley Christian, John Du Cane, Eddy Gary, Grace Kavadlo, Tamar Kaye, Erica Price, Johan Ringenbach, Monty Stillson & Annie Vo

EXTRA SPECIAL THANKS TO: Rosalie & Carl Kavadlo, John Du Cane, Grace Kavadlo, Adeline Kavadlo, Derek Brigham, Paul "Coach" Wade, Nick Collias, Chris Sainsbury at Crossfit Kingsboro, Mike Anderson, Annie Vo & Wilson Cash Kavadlo

The Kavadlo Brothers are contributors to Bodybuilding.com, where portions of this work have appeared.

– Table of Contents –

F O R E W O R D

By Jeff Cavaliere

When I was putting together a list of presenters that I wanted to speak at my annual live event in 2018, I knew I wanted to assemble a group of people that were not only knowledgeable in their field of expertise, but masters in it. My audience had been demanding that bodyweight training and calisthenics be one of the "must-have" topics. At that point, I knew who my "must-get" speaker would be: Al Kavadlo.

You see, what Al and his brother Danny did not know was that throughout the years, whenever I needed an additional resource for the proper way to perform, progress or regress a bodyweight exercise, I turned to them. Well, not literally. In this digital, on-demand world we live in, the answer to any question can be obtained within a few clicks of a mouse or a few strokes on a keyboard. Virtually any video or tutorial you need can be viewed from anywhere in the world on YouTube. That is where my education from these guys began.

But here's the thing.

Finding a video that addresses the questions you seek is not the challenge.

Finding someone you trust—and that's capable of delivering the right answers to those questions is much harder.

From the first video I watched, I knew who I'd be counting on to be my calisthenics resource.

You might be shocked to hear that it wasn't just the knowledge possessed by Al and Danny that kept me coming back to each new video. After all, my channel is known for putting the science into training and understanding not just "what" we're doing but "why" we're doing it. So how was that not the only thing that mattered to me at the end of the day?

Well, it's simple. Dating all the way back to grade school, I've found that there are two criteria beyond someone's grasp of the subject matter that can turn an average learning experience into something extraordinary and much more impactful: The first is a teacher that has a genuine desire to help—the type of person who lives to teach and would do it even if they weren't getting paid for it.

Hopefully, we've all been fortunate to have had at least one of them in our lifetime.

The teacher that stayed late, put in the extra time, and wouldn't consider their job done until they knew you understood everything. If you had one, you certainly remember them... and there's a reason for that—they cared about YOU and you knew it.

My second criteria is a teacher who teaches from experience. The very same experience that you're trying to understand at that moment. In other words, they've been where you've been and have now gotten to where you want to be. This makes that teacher not just able to relate to you better, but sympathetic to the challenges you're likely to face along the same bumpy road to mastery.

Heck, they have likely even failed at the same things you will find to be a struggle.

So what is so appealing about someone who has failed?

As the great Thomas Edison said, "Many of life's failures are people who did not realize how close they were to success when they gave up."

Persistence always wins.

And there is no way in the world that Al and Danny would have gotten to the level of mastery they have without being persistent, caring people.

They love to teach, live for challenges, and have learned their craft by refusing to accept failure as an option. What others might think is impossible, the Kavadlos see as something that will take just a little bit longer to achieve.

So whenever I am asked why, in a sea of so-called calisthenics experts, I choose Al and Danny Kavadlo as the gurus of my bodyweight gains, I come fully prepared to defend my choice because they make my decision so damn easy.

They are experts in their field. They care about helping me and every single person that wants to learn from them to achieve the same. Lastly, they possess the "in the trenches" experience that's been tested and mastered on themselves first, giving them a level of credibility and trustworthiness unable to be earned any other way.

As you're reading this, preparing to embark on or continue your bodyweight fitness journey, know that you are learning from the best. Al and Danny cut to a depth that most calisthenics practitioners will never reach. What you have before you is a well-researched, practical approach to achieving your fitness goals through bodyweight training, produced by the experts in their field.

Jeff Cavaliere MSPT, CSCS

ATHLEAN-X™

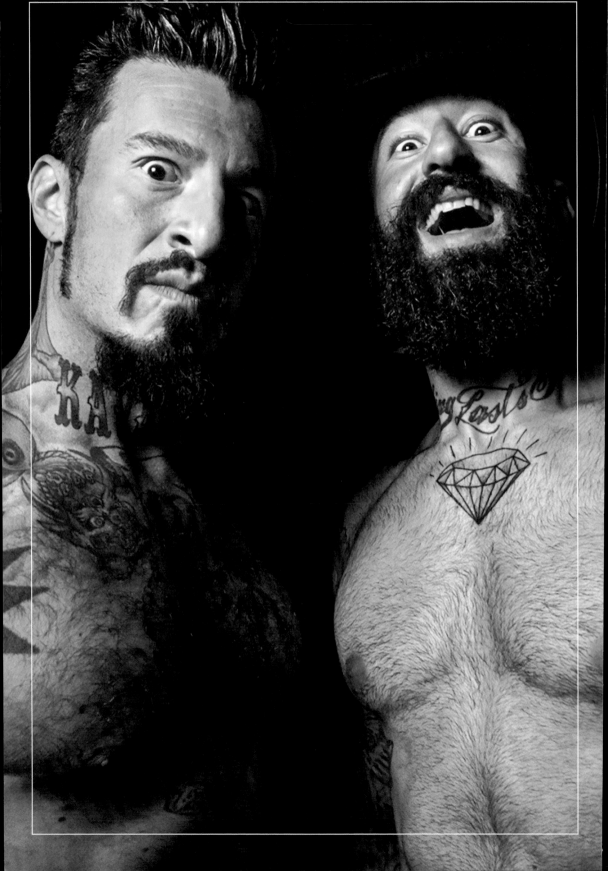

P R E F A C E

When we got started in fitness, we didn't have many options. We were just two broke kids from Brooklyn, so we began with what was available to us: push-ups and pull-ups. This was not because we were necessarily "calisthenics guys" but simply because we didn't have access to any equipment other than a basic doorway pull-up bar and the ground beneath our feet.

During the course of our journey, we would explore other methods of training. Once we were old enough to join a gym, free weights began to dominate our workouts. Though we never stopped doing push-ups and pull-ups, weight training had become the focus. We also experimented with machines, sandbags, medicine balls and everything else we could think of to maximize our strength gains. Additionally, as personal trainers in New York City, we wanted to familiarize ourselves with as many disciplines as possible so that we could provide the best service to all individuals.

Each of these modalities offers its own unique challenges and benefits. However, after years of experience with these different options, we eventually came full circle and returned to training with only our own bodyweight.

Pistol squats replaced barbell squats, L-sits replaced ab machines, handstand push-ups replaced military presses. The transition was so gradual that we hardly saw it coming. Little by little, we were slowly swapping out our favorite weight training exercises for their calisthenics counterparts. It is hard to say whether calisthenics chose us or we chose calisthenics.

Over the years, we have cultivated a following around the world for our unique style of bodyweight training, and we've been heralded for our ability to help our clients make maximal gains with minimal equipment.

We've written books about training with just a pull-up bar or no equipment at all. In **Street Workout** we even showed you how to make the world your gym.

In our previous release, **Get Strong**, we gave you our most stripped-down calisthenics program for building muscle and strength.

Although we have written extensively about bodyweight training, we still haven't covered it all. Not by a long shot. In fact, within the bodyweight kingdom there are two important pieces of apparatus which we've never addressed until now: rings and parallettes. We're still just getting started!

Whether this is your first Kavadlo Brothers book or your tenth, we're glad you're on this adventure with us. We're honored to be a part of your training and your life.

We're Working Out!   *Keep the Dream Alive!*

Al Kavadlo   Danny Kavadlo

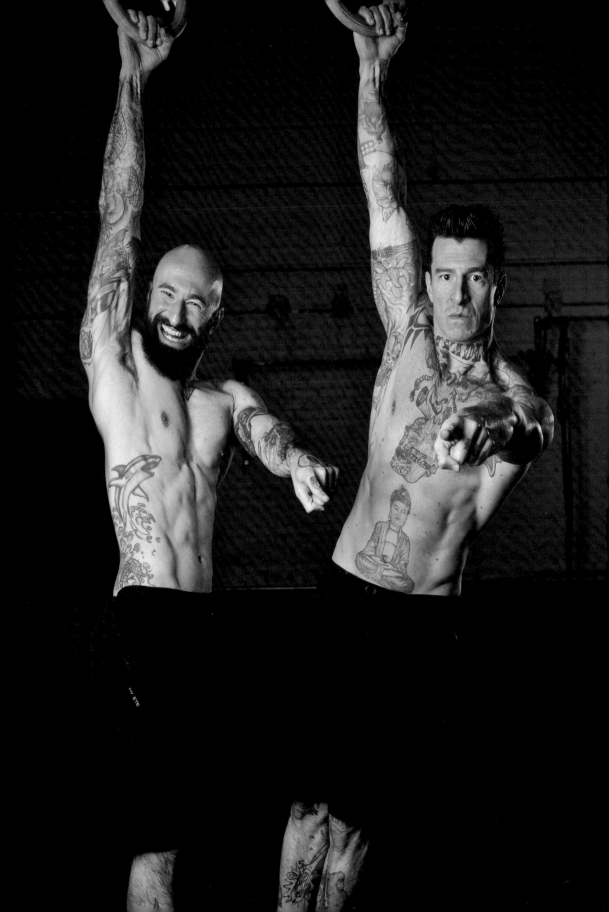

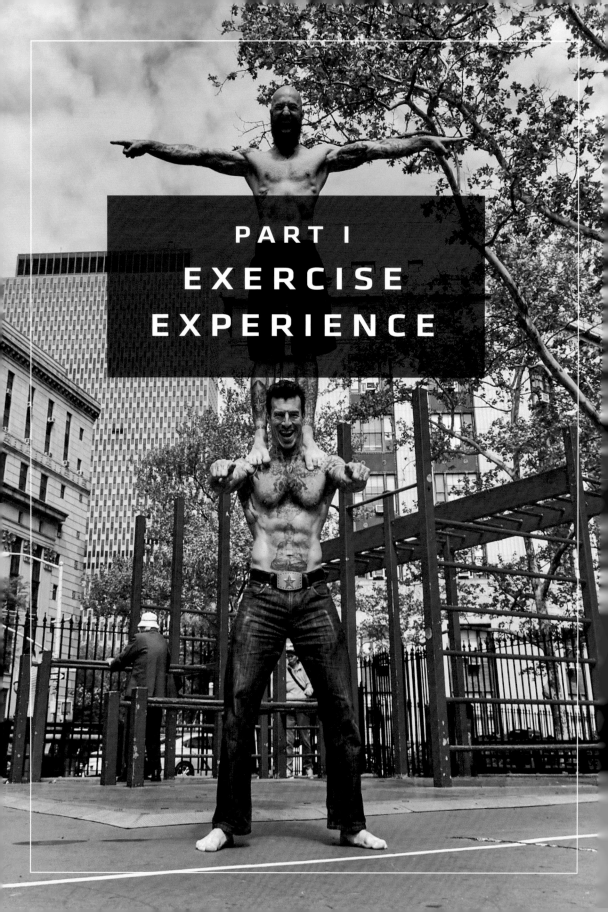

PART I
EXERCISE
EXPERIENCE

Take Action

In this life, there are many things which are out of our control. Thankfully, the decision to exercise is not one of them. By following this program, you can create the body that you seek, but you must be willing to take action and do the work.

Reading all the training books in the world will not teach you a single thing about working out if you do not embrace the practice. Exercise, like many things, must be experienced in order to be understood. No matter how helpful—and often necessary—having a guide may be, you will get more from traveling the terrain than from looking at the map. We can show you the path, but you must walk it alone.

When you devote your energy to things which you can control, you have a much greater chance of creating the life that you want. Success does not happen by accident. It is the result of your choices and actions. So don't be afraid to work hard in order to move forward.

WHY RINGS?

It's no secret that we're big fans of the pull-up bar. You can do a lot more with a simple straight bar than many people realize. And while many of the exercises in this book can also be done on a pull-up bar, there are numerous subtleties rendering them quite different on rings:

- Rings require extra core recruitment. Unlike a fixed pull-up bar, rings are free-floating and unstable. They can swing back and forth, rock side to side and even rotate. This forces your body to stabilize itself to a greater degree. As there is always a risk of injury when working with an unstable apparatus, be cautious and take your time.

- Because they are not connected to one another, rings allow you to pass in between them on moves like the skin-the-cat and muscle-up. Whereas you must maneuver around a pull-up bar, rings will not get in your way.

- Training with rings can potentially be more forgiving on your joints, particularly those of the wrists, shoulders and elbows. By allowing your hands to rotate, your joints may move in a more personalized range of motion.

- Though some exercises are more *challenging* when performed on rings, others are more *accessible*. It's a bit of a double-edged sword. Regardless, if you are used to training exclusively with a bar, those first few weeks of ring training may surprise you.

SUSPENSION TRAINERS ARE NOT RINGS!

As a general rule, we do not recommend using a suspension trainer (TRX) as a substitute for rings. Though some of these exercises can be done on a suspension trainer, others will not be possible due to the fact that suspension trainers fix both handles to a single point. The exercises in this book were designed for rings.

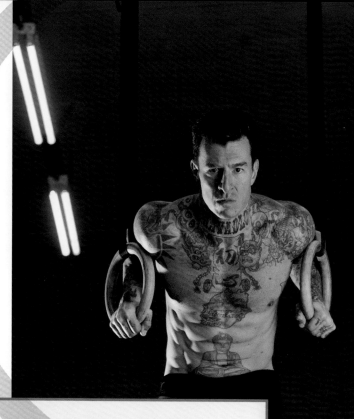

DIFFERENT TYPES OF RINGS

Wood - Natural feel, best grip

Metal - Most durable, most expensive, not as good for grip

Plastic - Durable, cheap, not as good for grip

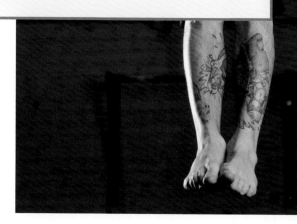

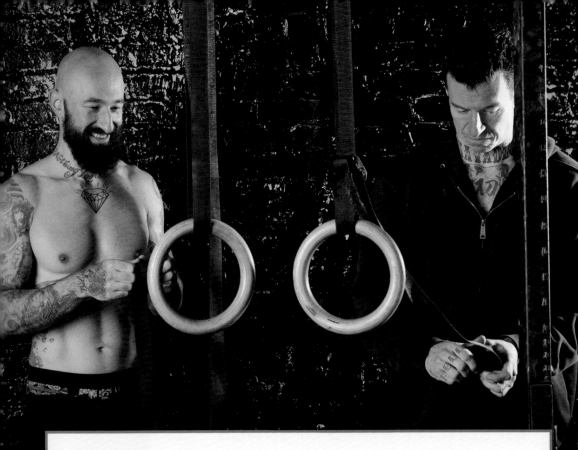

SETTING UP

✔ Some exercises require your rings to be set high enough to hang beneath them with your feet off the floor. (If your setup doesn't allow for this, just set your rings as high as possible.) Others will require the rings to be set just above waist height.

✔ Make sure your rings are the same height as one another.

✔ Set your rings approximately shoulder width apart and make sure that the straps are not twisted, and that they are threaded through the metal cams in the correct locking direction.

✔ Make sure the metal cams are substantially above your rings. If they are too low then your arms or wrists may rub against them.

✔ Double check that your rings are locked in place before putting your weight on them.

WHY PARALLETTES?

Parallel bars that are low to the ground are known as parallettes. Though they might not appear to offer anything special at first glance, these little, low bars are an amazing tool. Here's why:

- Wrist pain is one of the most common issues associated with floor exercises like planks, L-sits and handstands. Since parallettes allow your wrists to maintain a neutral position during these and other exercises, they offer a great way to work around (and possibly help eradicate) any issues that may plague your wrists.

- Squeezing parallettes while practicing these exercises creates more tension in your upper-body, which can facilitate a greater mind-muscle connection. This will help incur greater strength gains, especially with regard to your grip, core and shoulders.

- Elevating your hands with parallettes makes many exercises more accessible than when they're performed on the ground. Oftentimes, beginners lack flexibility and/or core strength. Having extra clearance beneath your body can make just enough of a difference to help you nail your first L-sit or tuck planche.

- You can adjust the width of your parallettes to suit your individual proportions, which you cannot do with affixed bars.

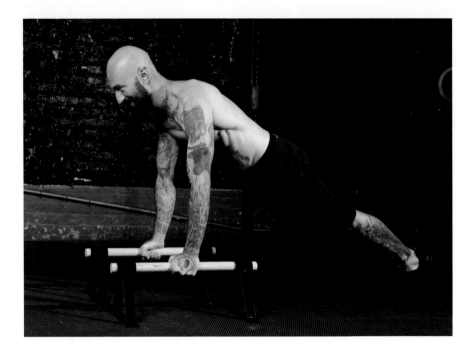

DUMBBELLS ARE NOT PARALLETTES!

As a general rule, we do not recommend using dumbbells or kettlebells as a substitute for parallettes. Though there are some exercises where they can be used (provided they are heavy enough), they are not ideal as they can compromise stability.

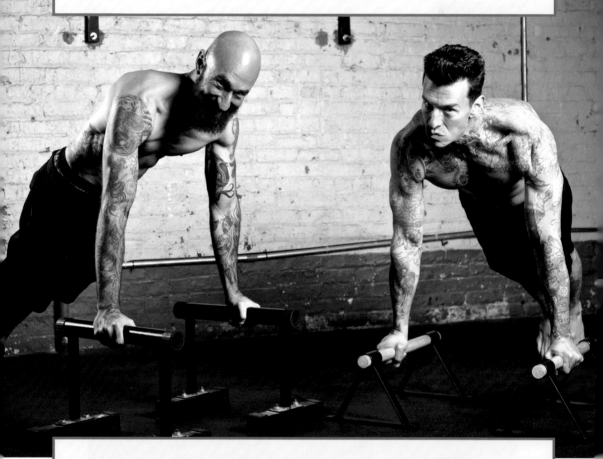

DIFFERENT TYPES OF PARALLETTES

Wood - Natural grip, good feel, durable, most expensive

Metal - Very durable, possibly heavy

PVC - Lightweight, less sturdy, least expensive

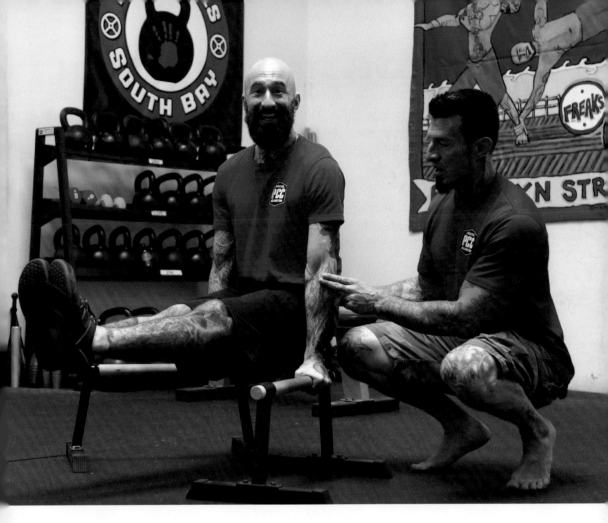

SETTING UP

✔ Use parallettes that are approximately 6-12 inches from the floor. Taller people will generally want to be a bit higher.

✔ Position the handles just outside of your hips. Be careful not to go too wide, as that may compromise your alignment and ability to create tension.

✔ Although traditional setups involve placing the bars parallel to one another, some will find it favorable to angle them slightly. Doing so can allow for better muscle activation in some instances.

THE NEXT LEVEL STRENGTH PROGRAM

The following program offers something for everyone. These workouts build strength, flexibility, control and body awareness. There is also a unique skill element to many of these exercises. To be clear, however, Next Level Strength is not gymnastics. Though some of these exercises may look like gymnastics movements, we are not competing with anyone but ourselves.

Next Level Strength is broken up into three levels, with each becoming progressively more difficult. As you advance, you will be met with more challenging exercise variations and increasingly demanding skills. You will also notice that there are more total exercises in the later levels. This is no accident. All three levels consist of workouts that gradually increase in training volume. This means you will slowly build up to more reps (or longer holds) of each movement over the course of several weeks. You need to add more total workout volume as well as more demanding exercises in order to continue to trigger further adaptations in your body.

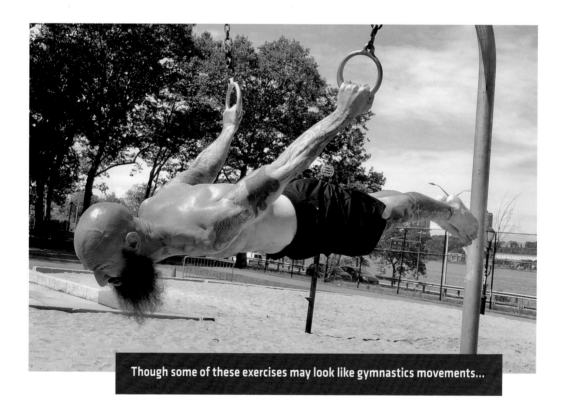

Though some of these exercises may look like gymnastics movements...

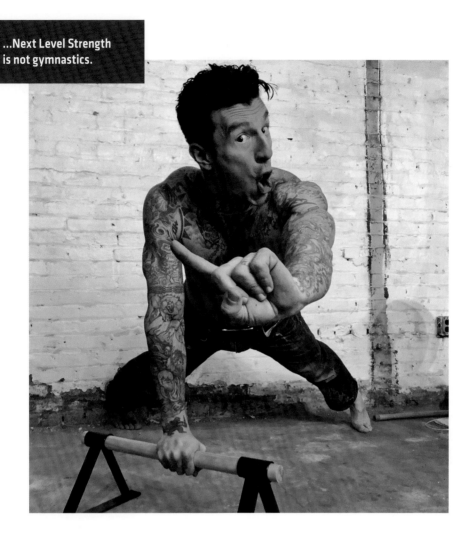

...Next Level Strength is not gymnastics.

During Level 1, you will do each workout 3-4 times a week for two weeks, with at least one day off in between training sessions. You will progress to a more challenging workout every two weeks. Following the program in this manner means you'll be devoting 8 weeks to this level, though some people will need more time, while others may need less. Each training session should not require more than 50 minutes of your time, and in many cases will require less. If you are a complete novice, we recommend taking your time with Level 1. You may even need more than eight weeks. There are also modifications which you can make to some of the Level 1 exercises to regress them if necessary. These are addressed in the "trainer talk" section of each exercise. Seasoned trainees who are new to rings and/or parallettes are encouraged to begin with Level 1 as well, as the specific demands of training with these apparatuses can take some getting used to.

In Level 2, you will follow a split routine. This means that your training will be split into two complementary workouts, both of which will be performed twice per week. The split routine allows for more total training volume without increasing the length of each individual training session. As with Level 1, you will progress to more challenging workouts every two weeks. Again, these workouts should not require more than 50 minutes of your time, and may require less. Experienced trainees may start right in with Level 2, provided they are able to pass the test at the end of Level 1.

In Level 3, you will also follow a split routine. As with the previous levels, you will progress to more challenging workouts every two weeks. Again, these workouts should not require more than 50 minutes of your time, and may require less. We do not recommend beginning at Level 3, regardless of your previous fitness background.

At the end of each level there is a test to determine whether or not you are ready to advance to the Next Level. If you pass the test, you move ahead. If not, then repeat the last two weeks and test again.

Remember, this program is the template, but you still need to deal with the reality of your situation. Always listen to your body and make adjustments based on what you are experiencing, even if that means deviating from the program as written.

Even after you've completed the final level, there are several "Next" Next Level exercises with which you can experiment. Your odyssey is not over until you decide you've gone as far as you're willing to go.

Let's take your strength to the Next Level!

GRIP TIPS

Rings - Standard Grip

1. Grab the rings with your thumbs wrapped around the opposite side as your fingers. Your thumbs should close on top of your other fingers.

2. Make sure your wrists remain in a neutral position; do not bend them back or flex them forward.

3. Squeeze the rings tightly with most of the weight in the upper part of your palms.

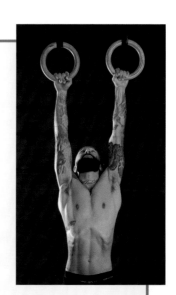

Rings - False Grip

1. Grab the rings with your thumbs wrapped around the opposite side as your fingers. Your thumbs should close on top of your other fingers.

2. Actively flex your hands in toward your wrists, choking as much of your hands as possible above the rings. The bone on the pinky side of your wrist should be in contact with the rings.

3. Squeeze the rings with most of the weight in the lower part of your palms.

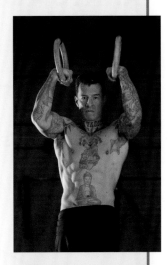

Rings - Support Grip

1. Grab the rings from above with your thumbs wrapped around the opposite side as your fingers. Your thumbs should close on top of your other fingers.

2. Keep your wrists as straight as possible with your arms close to your sides.

3. This is the grip you will use when you are positioned above the rings.

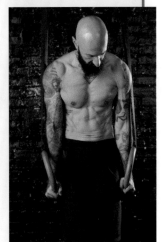

Parallettes - Standard Grip

1. Grab the bars with your hands parallel to one another and your elbow pits facing forward. Make sure your hands are in line with each other.

2. Make sure your wrists remain in a neutral position; do not let them bend backwards.

3. Squeeze the bars with your thumbs wrapped around the opposite side as your fingers.

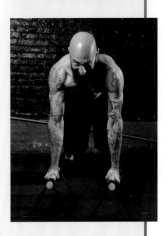

ANATOMY CHARTS

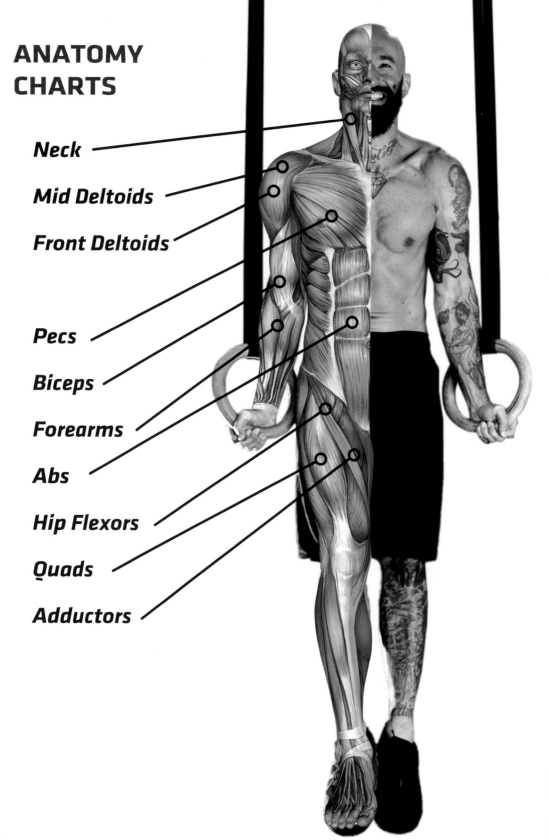

Neck

Mid Deltoids

Front Deltoids

Pecs

Biceps

Forearms

Abs

Hip Flexors

Quads

Adductors

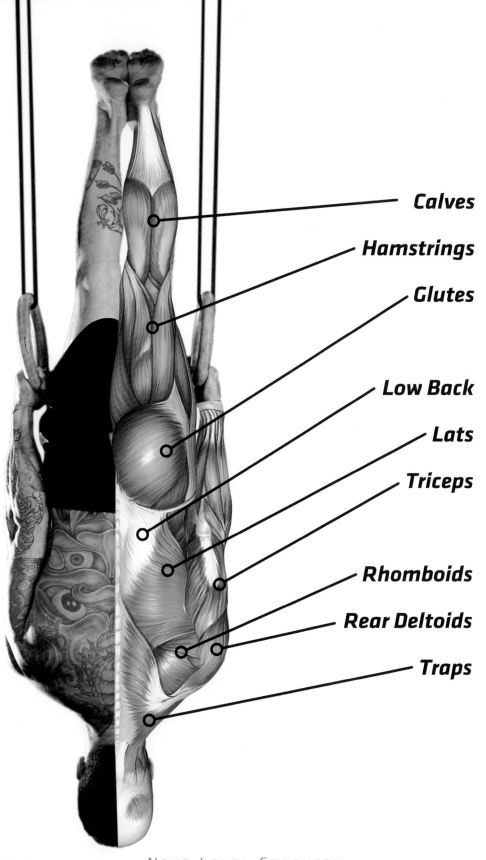

Calves

Hamstrings

Glutes

Low Back

Lats

Triceps

Rhomboids

Rear Deltoids

Traps

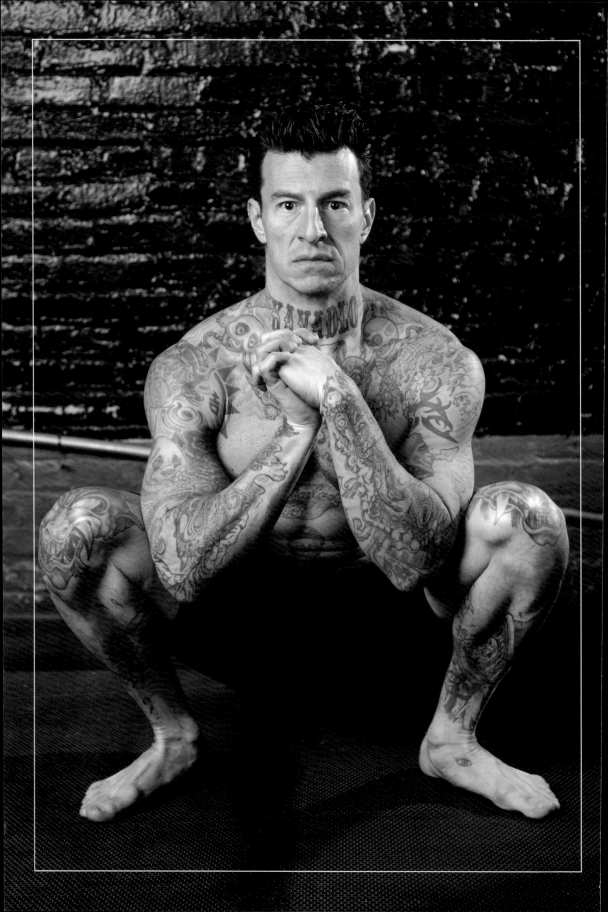

Warm-Ups

Use the following exercises to warm up your joints and muscles in preparation for what's ahead. You'll do these warm-ups throughout the entire program, so get familiar with them. You can also utilize them as a cool down at the end of the workout. Furthermore, we recommend doing these exercises throughout the day if you feel stiff or if you've been sedentary too long and need to move.

The warm-up is just as important as the rest of the workout, so take your time with these movements.

There are seven warm-ups included in this program: Neck Circle, Deep Squat Wrist Roll, The Titanic, Overhead Reach, Dead Hang, Elbow Corkscrew and Plank Knee Raise.

For each warm-up, we've included a three step description as well as "trainer talk" which provides further insight. Also included is a list of the muscles that are primarily emphasized. Be mindful, however, that all of the warm-ups employ the entire body to some degree.

Do each warm-up exercise for approximately 10 repetitions (on each side where applicable), or for 30 seconds in the case of static holds. Feel free to do certain warm-ups for longer if you see fit, based on your individual needs.

NECK CIRCLE

1. Turn your head all the way to the right and drop your chin toward your shoulder.

2. Rotate your chin toward your chest, then all the way to the left.

3. Continue rotating until you're looking up, then complete the circle by coming back to your right shoulder.

TRAINER TALK:

✓ Look in the direction that you are moving. Leading with your eyes can help you achieve a greater range of motion.

✓ Go slowly to avoid getting dizzy and make sure to repeat evenly in both directions.

Muscles Emphasized: Neck, Traps, Deltoids

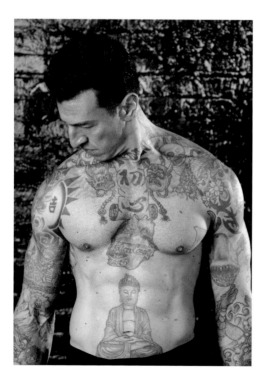
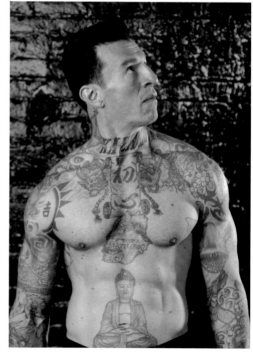

DEEP SQUAT WRIST ROLL

1. Assume a wide stance with your toes turned outward to approximately 45 degrees, then squat down as deep as you can without lifting your heels from the floor. You may need to flex your ankles and allow your knees to drift toward your toes in order to achieve full depth. Aim to touch your hamstrings against your calves.

2. Bring your elbows inside your hips and clasp your hands together with your fingers interlaced and palms facing each other.

3. Keep your arms relaxed in front of your chest as you begin to flex and extend your wrists in a circular motion, rolling your hands up, down, in and out. After several repetitions in both directions, reverse which hand is interlaced on top and repeat.

TRAINER TALK:

✔ Be careful not to let your knees cave inward. You can wedge your elbows against your knees to keep them in line with your feet.

Muscles Emphasized: Glutes, Hamstrings, Calves, Adductors, Forearms

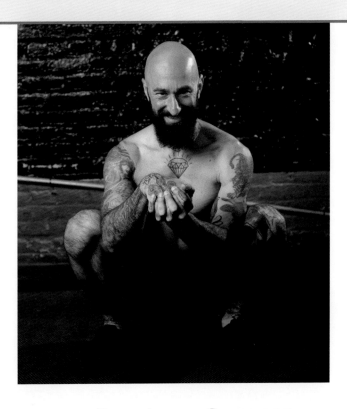

THE TITANIC

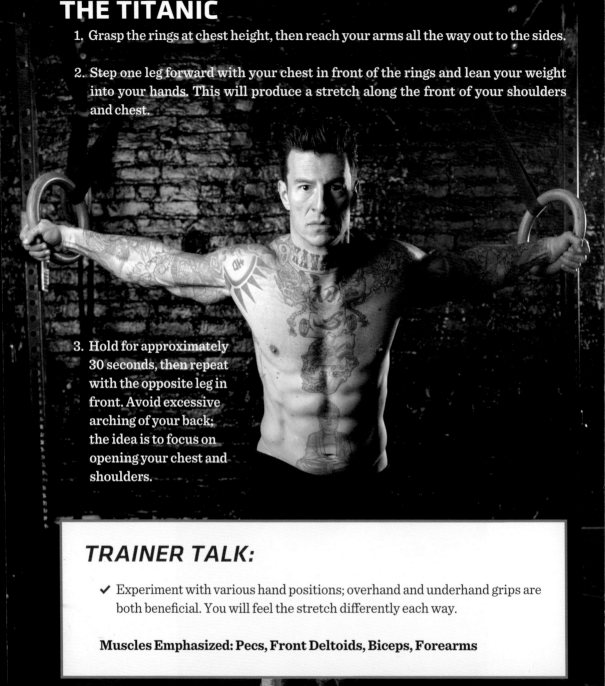

1. Grasp the rings at chest height, then reach your arms all the way out to the sides.

2. Step one leg forward with your chest in front of the rings and lean your weight into your hands. This will produce a stretch along the front of your shoulders and chest.

3. Hold for approximately 30 seconds, then repeat with the opposite leg in front. Avoid excessive arching of your back; the idea is to focus on opening your chest and shoulders.

TRAINER TALK:

✔ Experiment with various hand positions; overhand and underhand grips are both beneficial. You will feel the stretch differently each way.

Muscles Emphasized: Pecs, Front Deltoids, Biceps, Forearms

OVERHEAD REACH

1. Grasp the rings at chest height, then reach your arms all the way overhead.

2. Step one leg forward with your chest below your hands and lean your weight into your hands, producing a stretch along your upper back, shoulders and chest.

3. Hold for approximately 30 seconds, then repeat with the opposite leg in front. Avoid excessive arching of your back; the idea is to focus on opening your chest, shoulders and upper back.

TRAINER TALK:

✔ Experiment with various hand positions; overhand and underhand grips are both fair game. You will feel the stretch differently each way.

Muscles Emphasized: Lats, Pecs, Traps

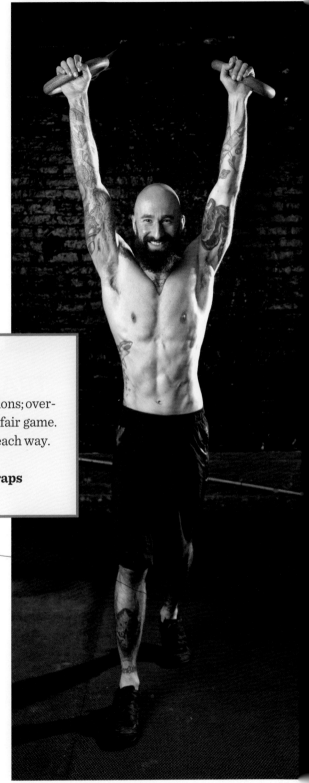

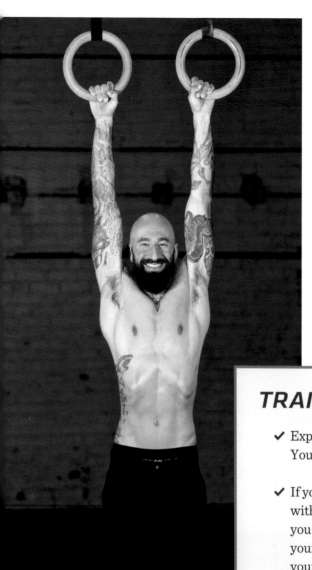

DEAD HANG

1. Set the rings overhead and grasp one in each hand with a standard grip, with your feet off the ground.

2. Allow your shoulders to relax and shrug upward. Every part of your body should be relaxed other than your grip. It may help to think about reaching your arms upward while simultaneously reaching your toes toward the floor.

3. Hold for approximately 30 seconds, breathing deeply and allowing your spine to decompress.

TRAINER TALK:

✔ Experiment with different head positions. You can look up, down or to the sides.

✔ If your rings aren't high enough to hang with your feet completely off the ground, you may rest your heels on the floor with your feet positioned slightly in front of your body.

Muscles Emphasized: Lats, Pecs, Deltoids, Forearms

ELBOW CORKSCREW

1. Stand with your feet wider than hip distance, then bend over and grasp your parallettes with your knees slightly bent.

2. Protract your shoulder blades away from each other and depress them down away from your ears. At the same time, squeeze the bars, extend your arms and turn your elbow pits as far forward as possible.

3. Relax briefly, allowing your shoulder blades to retract together while you rotate your elbow pits inward toward one another, then return to the previous position.

TRAINER TALK:

✔ Focus on the connection between your shoulder blades and your arms. Spreading your shoulder blades apart should flow seamlessly along with locking your elbows and turning your elbow pits forward.

✔ This position with your elbows locked, shoulder blades protracted and depressed, and elbow pits facing forward comes up often in parallette training. This exercise helps you learn how to properly engage the necessary muscles.

Muscles Emphasized: Triceps, Front Deltoids, Pecs, Rhomboids, Lats

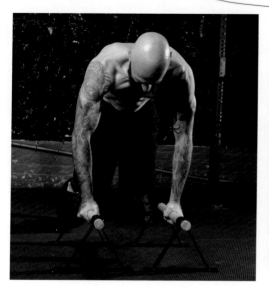 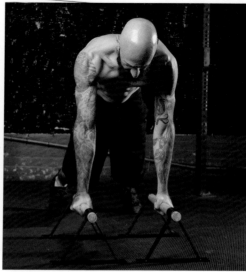

PLANK KNEE RAISE

1. Grasp your parallettes with your body fully extended and toes on the ground like the top of a push-up. Keep tension in your abs, legs and glutes while maintaining a straight line from your heels to the back of your head.

2. Carefully lift one leg in the air and raise your knee as far toward your chest as possible. Pause briefly with your foot still off the ground, and then return to the start position.

3. Repeat with the opposite leg, being mindful to stay in complete control of your movement.

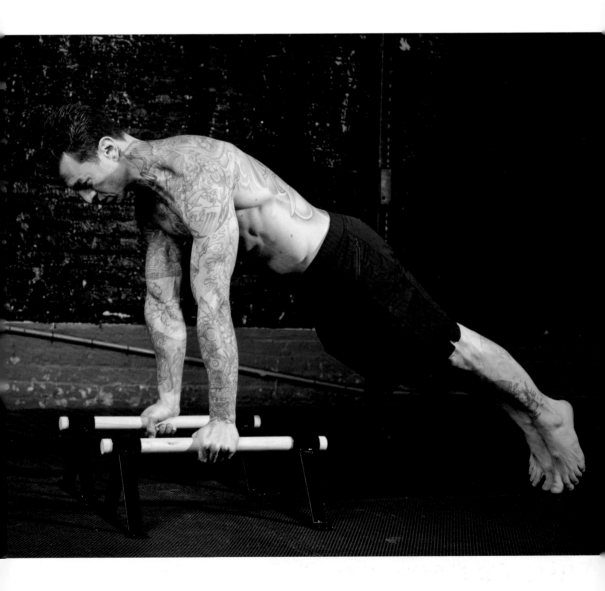

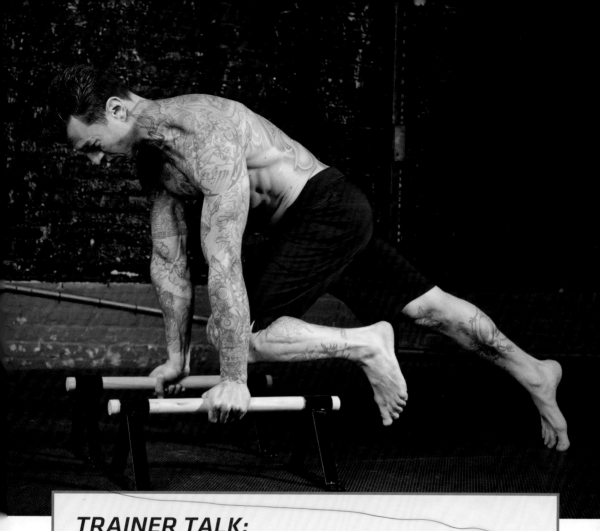

TRAINER TALK:

✔ You might be surprised by how much you feel your abs the first time you try this exercise. Anytime you remove a contact point during a plank, your abs will have to pick up the slack.

Muscles Emphasized: Abs, Hip Flexors, Pecs, Front Deltoids, Triceps

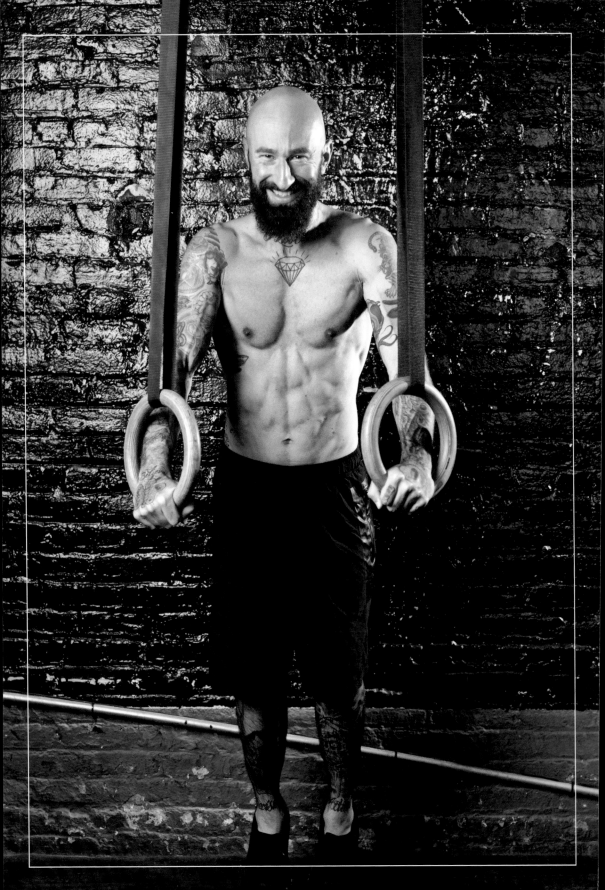

LEVEL 1

Unstoppable

This is the starting point from which you will build your base of strength and control. Stay on this level for eight weeks, gradually increasing the amount of reps performed on each exercise every two weeks as described in the programming ahead.

There are seven exercises in Level 1: Table Bridge to Grounded L-sit, N-sit, Bodyweight Row, High Rings Push-up, Flex Hang/Negative Pull-up, Hanging Knee Raise and Rings Assisted Squat.

For each exercise, we've included a three-step description as well as "trainer talk" which provides further insight. Also included is a list of the muscles that are primarily emphasized. Be mindful, however, that all of these exercises employ the entire body to some degree.

After the exercises, there are charts containing specific program details including sets, reps and rest times. When you reach the end, there is a test to determine if you are ready to progress to the Next Level.

TABLE BRIDGE TO GROUNDED L-SIT

1. Grab your parallettes with your hands beneath your shoulders and your hips and feet several inches in front of your hands. Your feet will be flat on the ground.

2. Press your feet into the floor, raising your hips into the air so that you form a straight line from your knees to your shoulders. Dr op your head back and pause briefly.

3. Lower your hips down, straighten your legs and allow your feet to roll up so that only the backs of your heels remain in contact with the floor. Your hips will slide back beneath your shoulders and you will wind up in an L-sit position with your heels resting on the floor. Pause briefly, then return to the bridge position. You can experiment with pointing or flexing your feet to find what works best for you.

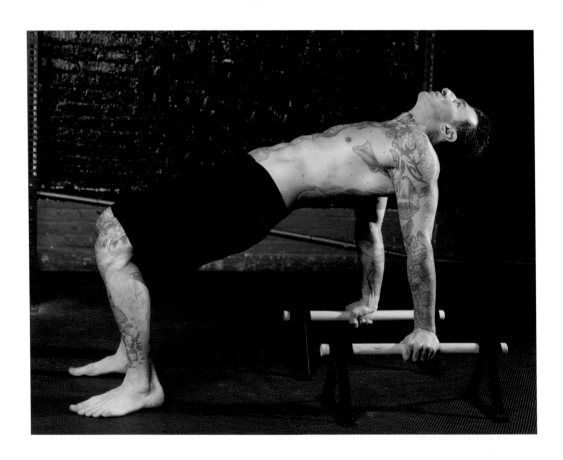

TRAINER TALK:

- ✔ It's okay in the beginning to use some momentum to switch from the bridge to the grounded L-sit, though ultimately we encourage you to go slowly.

- ✔ Experiment with how far your feet are from your hands. The closer your feet are to your hands, the more difficult the exercise becomes, so feel free to start with your heels fairly far from your body at first.

Muscles Emphasized: Hamstrings, Glutes, Abs, Deltoids, Triceps

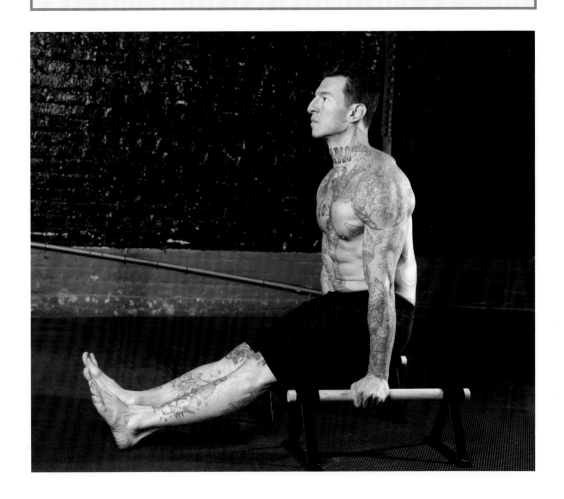

N-SIT

1. Grab your parallettes with your torso upright and your shoulders and hips directly above your hands. Your feet will be flat on the floor with your knees bent.

2. Press down into the handles, point your elbow pits forward and allow your upper back to round slightly so that you can spread your shoulder blades apart, being mindful not to let your shoulders shrug up toward your ears.

3. Lift your feet off the floor, bringing your knees toward your chest with your heels beneath them so that your body resembles a capital letter "N". Hold this position. You can experiment with pointing or flexing your feet to find what works best for you.

TRAINER TALK:

✔ If you aren't able to perform the exercise with both feet off the ground, you can try lifting just one foot.

✔ You may find yourself swinging or shaking a bit on your first attempts. This is normal and should minimize with practice.

Muscles Emphasized: Abs, Hip Flexors, Pecs, Lats, Deltoids, Triceps

---

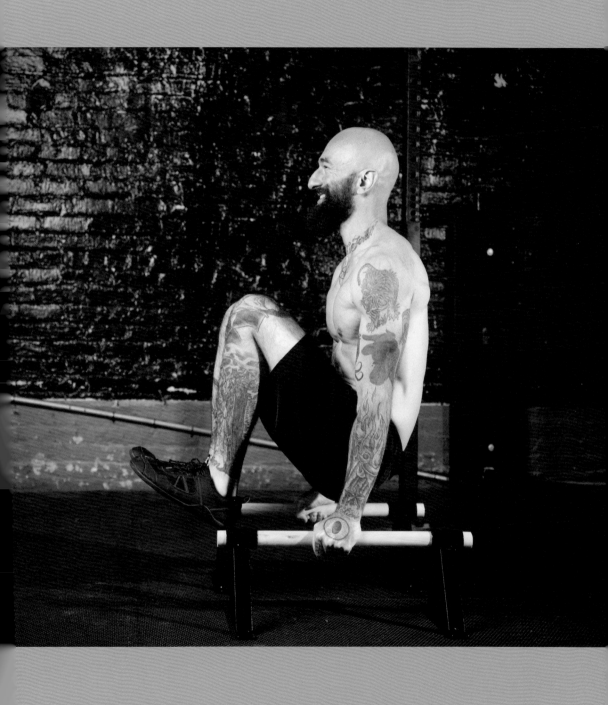

BODYWEIGHT ROW

1. Set your rings to approximately hip height. Grab one ring in each hand with a standard grip, then lean your body back at a 45 degree angle to the floor, forming a straight line from your heels to the back of your head. This will be your starting position. You can try palms facing toward one another, palms facing up or palms facing down. Each position will place a slightly different emphasis on the muscles.

2. Keeping your whole body engaged, pull your chest up toward your wrists, squeezing your shoulder blades toward each other on the way up. Be mindful not to let your shoulders shrug up toward your ears as you pull.

3. Lower back to the start position, allowing your shoulder blades to spread apart at the bottom.

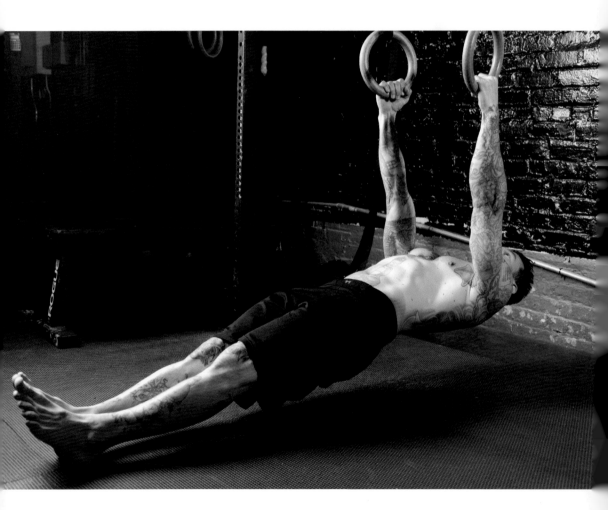

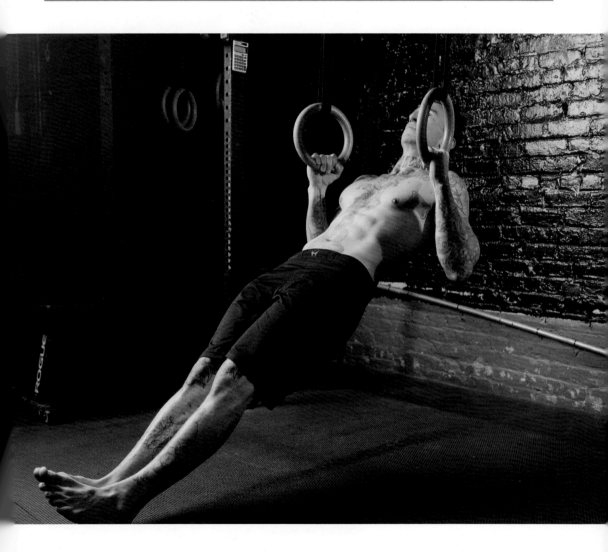

HIGH RINGS PUSH-UP

1. Set your rings to approximately hip height. Grab one ring in each hand from above, keeping your toes on the ground. Back your feet up so that you form a straight line from your heels to the back of your head. Your body should be at approximately a 45 degree angle from the ground. This will be your starting position. You can try palms facing toward one another or palms facing down. Each position will place a slightly different emphasis on the muscles.

2. Keeping your whole body engaged, lower your chest toward your hands, allowing your shoulder blades to retract toward each other on the way down.

3. Carefully press yourself back to the start position, spreading your shoulder blades apart as your ascend. Be mindful not to let your shoulders shrug up toward your ears.

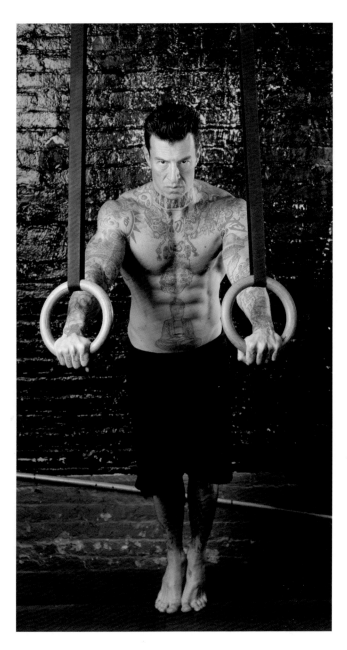

TRAINER TALK:

- ✔ If you aren't able to perform the exercise properly, try positioning your rings a bit higher for better leverage.

- ✔ You may find yourself swinging or shaking a bit on your first attempts. This is normal and should minimize with practice.

**Muscles Emphasized:
Pecs, Front Deltoids,
Triceps, Abs**

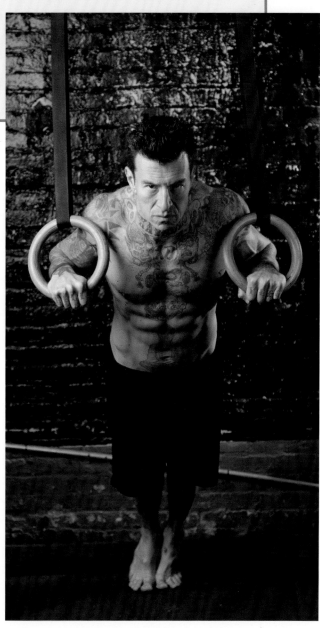

FLEX HANG/NEGATIVE PULL-UP

1. Stand on an elevated surface and grab one ring in each hand with a standard, under-hand grip.

2. With your arms bent and your chin above the rings, hug your hands toward your chest, tense your midsection and carefully step your feet off of the surface, maintaining a flexed-arm position.

3. Hold, then carefully lower yourself down until your arms are straight before coming off the rings. Be mindful not to let your shoulders shrug up toward your ears during the negative. You may find yourself swinging or shaking a bit on your first attempts. This is normal and should minimize with practice.

TRAINER TALK:

✔ Aim to perform your negative at a consistent pace. It's common to drop too quickly during the second half of the lowering phase, so be extra careful to go slowly from the time you reach a 90 degree angle at your elbows until you are in a dead hang.

✔ Though you will begin in an underhand position, allow your hands to rotate outward as you descend.

Muscles Emphasized: Lats, Pecs, Rear Deltoids, Rhomboids, Biceps, Abs

---

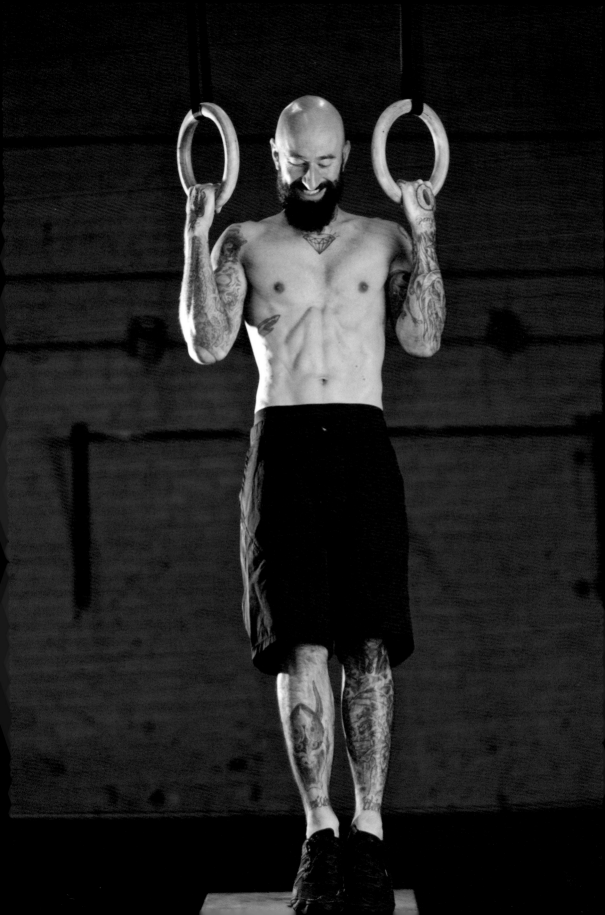

HANGING KNEE RAISE

1. Set the rings overhead and grasp one in each hand with a standard overhand grip. Your feet should be slightly off the ground in front of your body.

2. Keep your elbows locked as you lift your knees toward your chest, tilting your pelvis slightly forward at the top in order to fully engage your abs.

3. Lower your legs back to the bottom, being mindful not to pick up momentum on the way down. Do your best to minimize any swinging, but a small amount may be unavoidable. Remember, your feet should remain slightly in front of your body in the bottom position.

TRAINER TALK:

✔ If you aren't able to raise your knees all the way to your chest, you can start with a partial range of motion.

Muscles Emphasized: Abs, Hip Flexors, Lats, Forearms

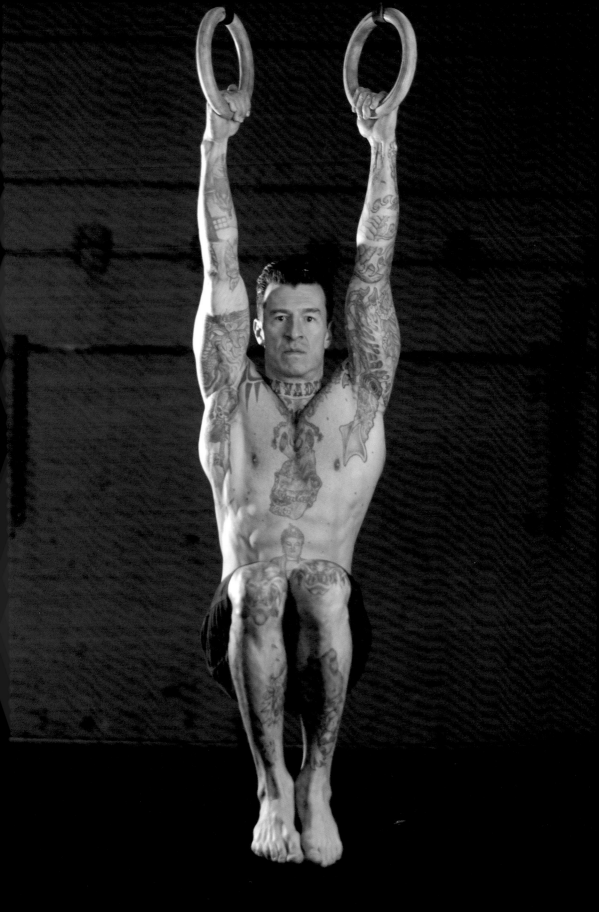

RINGS ASSISTED SQUAT

1. Stand up straight with your feet approximately shoulder width apart, holding one ring in each hand at approximately chest height. Experiment with different foot positions. Some people feel better with their toes turned out, while others prefer to keep their feet parallel.

2. Reach your arms forward and bend from your hips, knees and ankles, lowering until your hamstrings make contact with your calves. Keep your heels flat on the ground the entire time.

3. Pause briefly at the bottom before standing back up to the top position, gently pulling on the rings for assistance as needed.

TRAINER TALK:

✔ If you aren't able to lower yourself all the way down without your heels coming up, you may start with a partial range of motion.

✔ Rely on your arms only as needed, doing the majority of the work with your legs.

Muscles Emphasized: Quadriceps, Hamstrings, Glutes, Calves

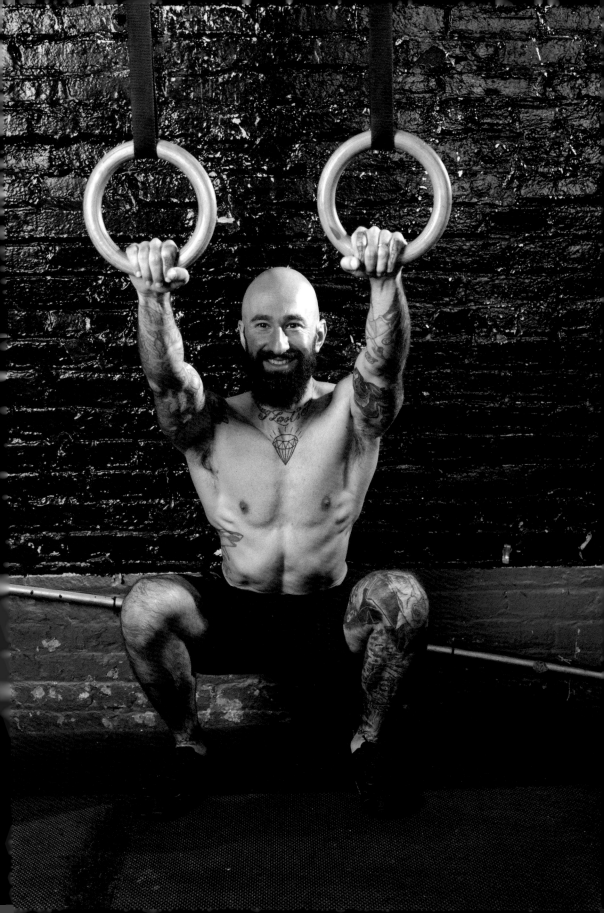

LEVEL 1—WEEKS 1 AND 2

✔ Repeat this workout 3-4 times a week for the next two weeks with at least one day off between each session.

✔ Following the warm-up described earlier, perform all exercises in sequence as written, resting for approximately 60-90 seconds between each set.

✔ Perform all reps with a controlled cadence and full range of motion.

✔ If you fail to complete the total necessary reps, you may add additional sets in order to get them finished.

✔ Do not move on until you can complete this workout as written. If you cannot do so, then continue to repeat this workout for as many weeks as necessary until you can.

Table Bridge to Grounded L-sit...............3 sets x 3 reps

N-sit..3 sets x 5 second hold

Bodyweight Row ....3 sets x 5 reps

High Rings Push-up ....3 sets x 5 reps

Flex Hang/Negative Pull-up....................3 sets x 5 second hold + 5 second negative

Hanging Knee Raise...................................3 sets x 5 reps

Rings Assisted Squat................................3 sets x 10 reps

LEVEL 1—WEEKS 3 AND 4

✔ Repeat this workout 3-4 times a week for the next two weeks with at least one day off between each session.

✔ Following the warm-up described earlier, perform all exercises in sequence as written, resting for approximately 60-90 seconds between each set.

✔ Perform all reps with a controlled cadence and full range of motion.

✔ If you fail to complete the total necessary reps, you may add additional sets in order to get them finished.

✔ Do not move on until you can complete this workout as written. If you cannot do so, then continue to repeat this workout for as many weeks as necessary until you can.

Table Bridge to Grounded L-sit...............3 sets x 5 reps

N-sit...3 sets x 10 second hold

Bodyweight Row ....3 sets x 8 reps

High Rings Push-up ....3 sets x 8 reps

Flex Hang/Negative Pull-up ....3 sets x 10 second hold +
                                                                        5 second negative

Hanging Knee Raise..................................3 sets x 8 reps

Rings Assisted Squat.................................3 sets x 15 reps

LEVEL 1—WEEKS 5 AND 6

✔ Repeat this workout 3-4 times a week for the next two weeks with at least one day off between each session.

✔ Following the warm-up described earlier, perform all exercises in sequence as written, resting for approximately 60-90 seconds between each set.

✔ Perform all reps with a controlled cadence and full range of motion.

✔ If you fail to complete the total necessary reps, you may add additional sets in order to get them finished.

✔ Do not move on until you can complete this workout as written. If you cannot do so, then continue to repeat this workout for as many weeks as necessary until you can.

Table Bridge to Grounded L-sit .... 3 sets x 6 reps

N-sit .... 3 sets x 15 second hold

Bodyweight Row .... 3 sets x 10 reps

High Rings Push-up .... 3 sets x 10 reps

Flex Hang/Negative Pull-up .... 3 sets x 10 second hold +
10 second negative

Hanging Knee Raise .... 3 sets x 10 reps

Rings Assisted Squat .... 3 sets x 20 reps

LEVEL 1—WEEKS 7 AND 8

✔ Repeat this workout 3-4 times a week for the next two weeks with at least one day off between each session.

✔ Following the warm-up described earlier, perform all exercises in sequence as written, resting for approximately 60-90 seconds between each set.

✔ Perform all reps with a controlled cadence and full range of motion.

✔ If you fail to complete the total necessary reps, you may add additional sets in order to get them finished.

✔ Do not move on until you can complete this workout as written. If you cannot do so, then continue to repeat this workout for as many weeks as necessary until you can.

✔ Once you can complete this workout as written, take the Level 1 Test to see if you are ready to advance to the Next Level.

Table Bridge to Grounded L-sit...............3 sets x 8 reps

N-sit..3 sets x 20 second hold

Bodyweight Row ....3 sets x 12 reps

High Rings Push-up ....3 sets x 12 reps

Flex Hang/Negative Pull-up...................3 sets x 15 second hold +
10 second negative

Hanging Knee Raise...................................3 sets x 12 reps

Rings Assisted Squat.................................2 sets x 30 reps

LEVEL 1–TEST

If you can complete the following workout in sequence with less than 60 seconds between each exercise, then move onto Level 2 the following week. If you cannot complete the test, repeat the last two weeks of training, then test yourself again in two weeks.

You may choose to do the test in place of your final training day of week 8 or you may do it as the first day of the following week. Either way, give yourself two full days off from any formal strength training before and after attempting this test.

TAKE TWO FULL DAYS REST BEFORE THIS TEST

- ✔ Table Bridge to Grounded L-sit..............10 reps
- ✔ N-sit ....30 second hold
- ✔ Bodyweight Row ....15 reps
- ✔ High Rings Push-up....................................15 reps
- ✔ Flex Hang/Negative Pull-up ....20 second hold + 10 second negative
- ✔ Hanging Knee Raise ....15 reps
- ✔ Rings Assisted Squat.................................40 reps

TAKE LEVEL 1 TEST

DID YOU PASS?

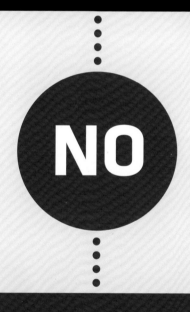

NO

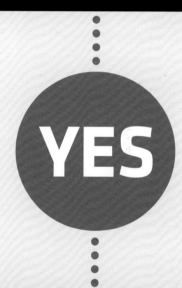

YES

GO BACK TO LEVEL 1 WEEK 7

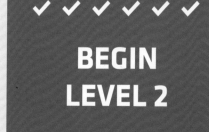

BEGIN LEVEL 2

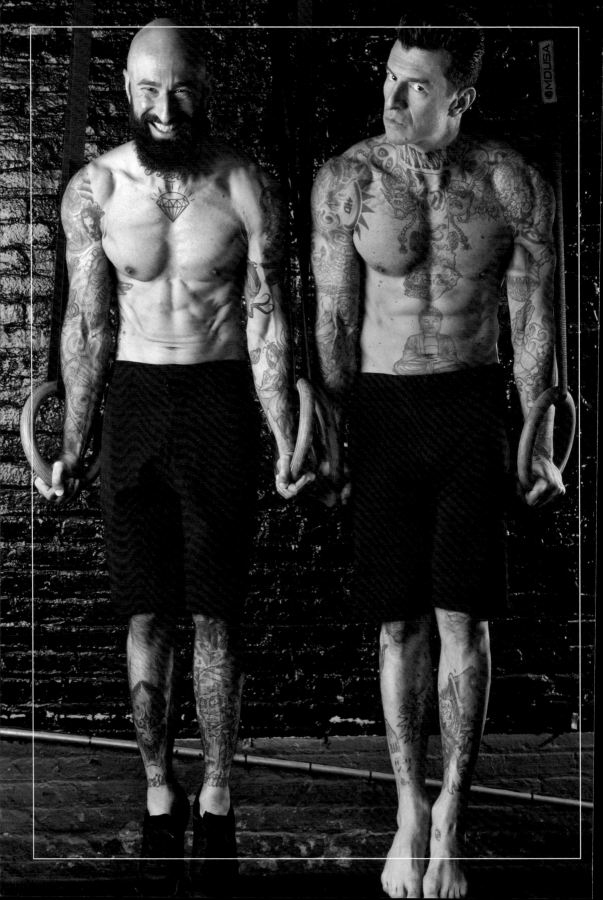

LEVEL 2

Unbreakable

Now that you have established a solid foundation, you are ready to advance to more difficult exercise progressions. You will also continue to practice some of the exercises from Level 1 in this phase of your training.

Stay on this level for eight weeks, gradually increasing the number of reps performed on each exercise every two weeks as described in the programming ahead.

There are ten new exercises in Level 2: Jump Through, L-sit, Planche Lean, Pike Press, Pull-up, Support Hold, Inverted Hang, False Grip Flex Hang/Negative Pull-up, Rings Assisted Archer Squat and Rings Assisted Pistol Squat.

For each new exercise, we've included a three-step description as well as "trainer talk" which provides further insight. Also included is a list of the muscles that are primarily emphasized. Be mindful, however, that all of these exercises employ the entire body to some degree.

After the exercises, there are charts containing specific program details including sets, reps and rest times. When you reach the end of this section there is a test to determine if you are ready to progress to the Next Level.

JUMP THROUGH

1. Grasp your parallettes with your body fully extended and toes on the ground, forming a straight line from your heels to the back of your head, like the top of a push-up.

2. Without moving your hands, actively press into the parallettes with your arms. Jump forward and slide your body through to the other side. You will wind up in an upside-down plank position with your chest facing upward.

3. Drag your heels backward slightly, then jump yourself back through to the other side, returning to the standard push-up position. That's one rep.

TRAINER TALK:

✔ When you are in the reverse plank phase of the movement, focus on pushing your chest all the way up and out while actively squeezing your legs and glutes to get the most from the exercise.

✔ Your first several attempts might feel awkward. Keep practicing.

Muscles Emphasized: Pecs, Triceps, Front Deltoids, Low Back, Hamstrings, Glutes, Quads

---

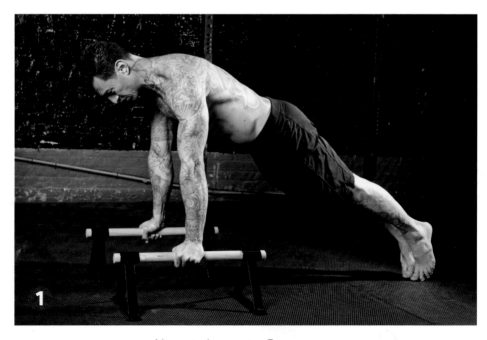

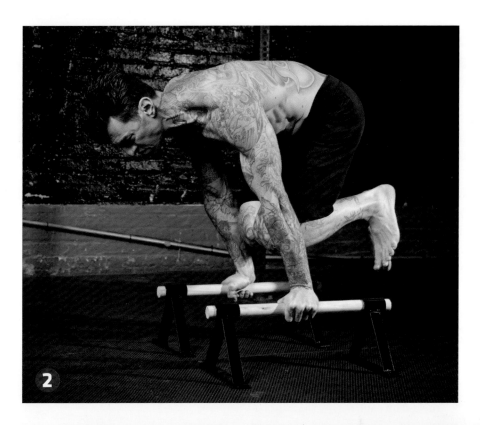

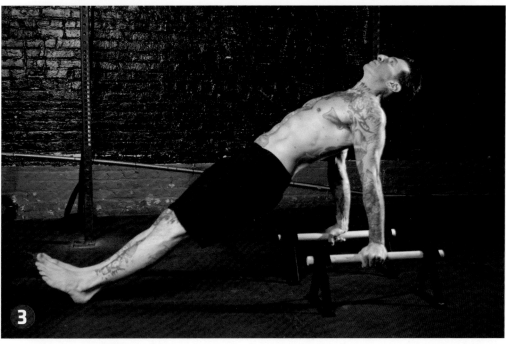

L-SIT

1. Grab your parallettes with your torso upright and your shoulders and hips directly above your hands. Your feet will be flat on the floor with your knees bent.

2. Press down into the handles, point your elbow pits forward and allow your upper back to round slightly so that you can spread your shoulder blades apart, being mindful not to let your shoulders shrug up toward your ears.

3. Lift your feet off the floor and extend your legs away from your body until they are parallel to the ground. Your body will resemble a capital letter "L". You may point or flex your toes. Either way make sure your feet remain engaged. You may find yourself swinging or shaking a bit on your first attempts. This is normal and should minimize with practice.

TRAINER TALK:

✔ If you aren't able to perform the exercise with both legs fully extended, you can try keeping one leg tucked and one leg straight. Alternate which leg is tucked on each set.

✔ You may need to position your hips behind your hands at first, though with practice, you should be able to keep them directly in line with your hands.

Muscles Emphasized: Abs, Pecs, Triceps, Lats, Deltoids, Hip Flexors, Quads

---

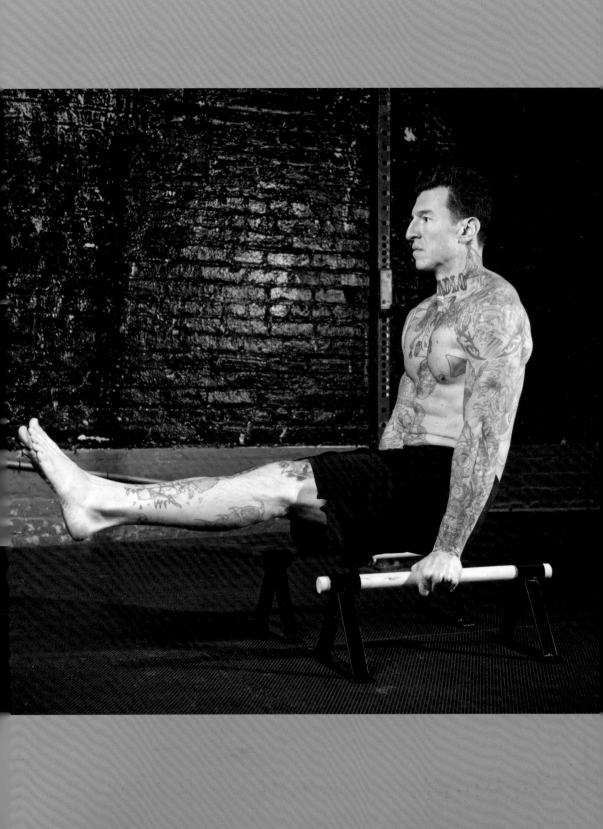

PLANCHE LEAN

1. Grasp your parallettes with your hands positioned directly beneath your shoulders and your body in a straight line from the back of your head to your heels.

2. Keep your hands in place and walk your toes forward, allowing your shoulders to drift in front of your hands.

3. Spread your shoulder blades apart, lock your elbows, press your hands into the bars and hold this position. There is a good deal of wrist mobility required to achieve a deep planche lean.

TRAINER TALK:

✔ The farther forward your shoulders wind up, the more difficult the exercise becomes. Experiment with finding your threshold point, then gradually work toward pushing it further.

Muscles Emphasized: Pecs, Front Deltoids, Triceps, Abs

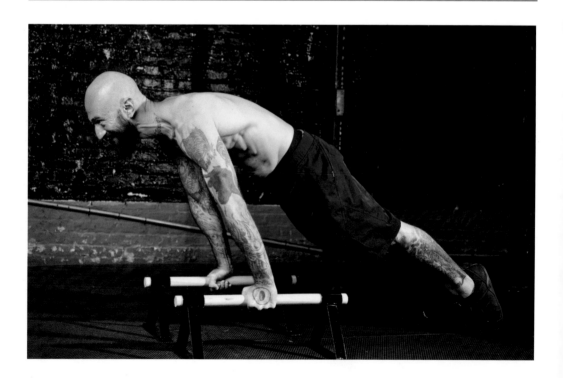

PIKE PRESS

1. Stand with your feet slightly wider than hip distance, then bend over and grasp your parallettes. Keep your hips in the air above your hands.

2. Look in front of your hands, bend your arms and lower your head toward the ground. Keep your elbows relatively close to your sides. Do not allow them to flare out.

3. Pause briefly before your head touches the ground, then press yourself back to the top.

TRAINER TALK:

✔ You may feel a deep stretch in your hamstrings during this exercise. If you cannot maintain straight legs, you may allow a slight bend in your knees in order to preserve the rest of your alignment.

✔ If you aren't able to lower yourself all the way down, you may start with a partial range of motion.

Muscles Emphasized: Deltoids, Traps, Pecs, Triceps

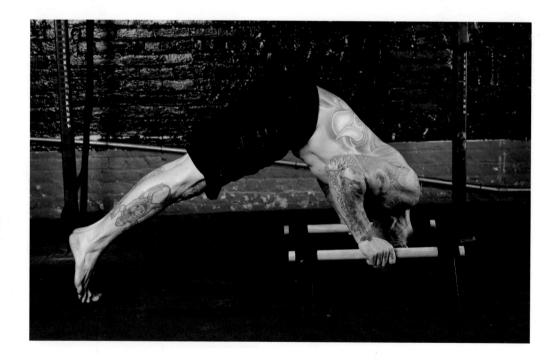

PULL-UP

1. Set the rings overhead and grasp one in each hand with a standard overhand grip and your feet off the ground.

2. Keep your abs braced and your legs straight as you begin pulling your hands toward your shoulders while driving your elbows down to your hips. Don't bend your knees or swing your legs.

3. When your chin is higher than your knuckles, carefully lower back to the bottom position.

TRAINER TALK:

✔ Allow your hands to rotate as you pull. Though you will begin in an overhand grip, most people will find that their hands naturally rotate to an underhand (or partially under-hand) position at the top.

✔ Keep your body as stable as possible. Do your best to avoid using any momentum.

Muscles Emphasized:
Lats, Pecs, Rear Deltoids,
Rhomboids, Biceps, Abs

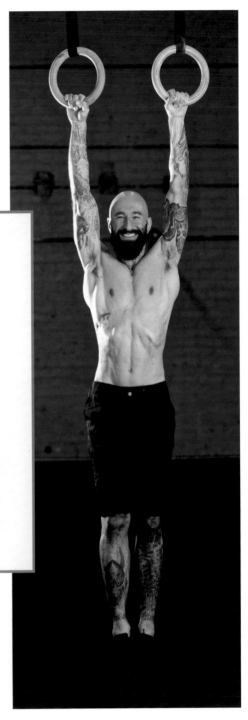

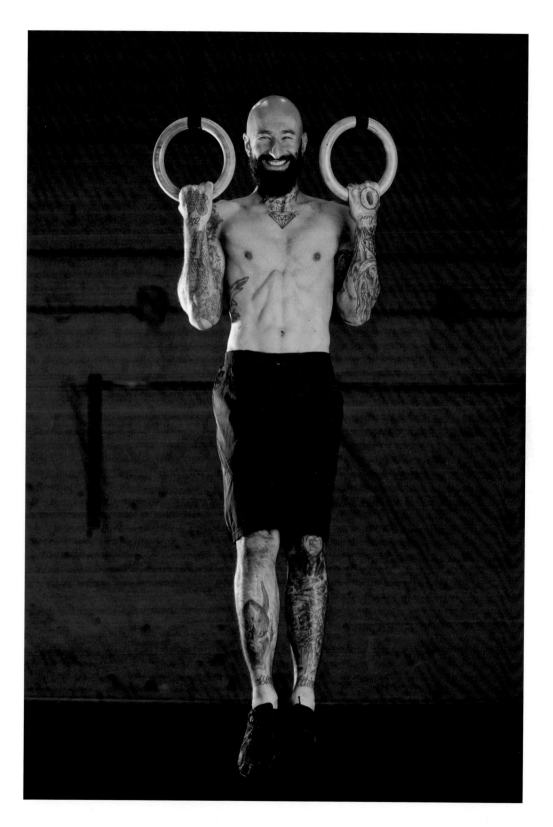

SUPPORT HOLD

1. Position your rings at approximately chest height and grab one ring in each hand.

2. Jump into an upright position above the rings and lock your elbows completely with your hands close to your sides.

3. Keep your feet slightly in front of your hips. As you begin to fatigue, think about actively pressing your hands and arms into the rings to stay in position. You may also experiment with rotating your palms forward for an added challenge.

TRAINER TALK:

✔ Newcomers to this exercise are often surprised by how challenging it can be to simply support your body upright above the rings. If you aren't able to hold the position at first, you may regress the exercise by resting one or both feet on an elevated surface for assistance.

Muscles Emphasized: Traps, Lats, Pecs, Deltoids, Triceps, Abs

---

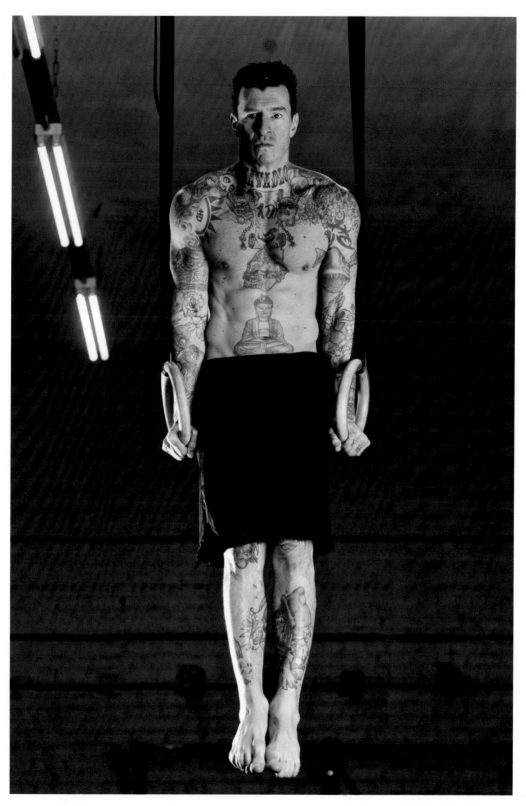

NEXT LEVEL STRENGTH

INVERTED HANG

1. Set the rings overhead and grasp one in each hand with a standard overhand grip.

2. Pull your knees toward your chest and lean your torso back by dragging your hands down toward your hips in a straight arm pull.

3. Reach your feet and legs over your head, extending your body until you are completely upside-down. Hold this position, then come down as carefully as possible. You can think of this exercise as an upside-down version of the support hold.

TRAINER TALK:

✔ In addition to the strength component, there is a tremendous spacial aware-ness element to this exercise. Try not to get discouraged if you're thrown by this on your initial attempts.

✔ At first it will be helpful to look toward your toes while you are inverted in order to make sure your body is in a straight line. Once you are balanced, you can experiment with looking out ahead instead.

Muscles Emphasized: Traps, Deltoids, Abs, Glutes, Forearms

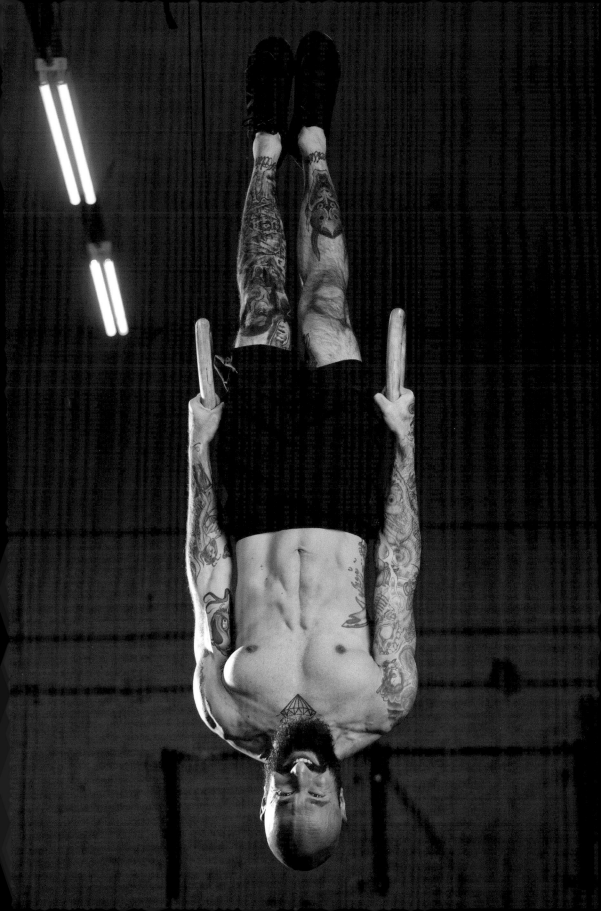

FALSE GRIP FLEX HANG/
NEGATIVE PULL-UP

1. Stand on an elevated surface and grab one ring in each hand using a false grip.

2. With your arms bent and your chin above the rings, hug your hands toward your chest, tense your midsection and carefully step your feet off of the surface, maintaining a flexed-arm position.

3. Hold here, then carefully lower yourself down until your arms are straight before coming off the rings. Be mindful not to let your shoulders shrug up toward your ears during the negative. You may find yourself losing your false grip a bit on your first attempts. This is normal and will improve with practice.

TRAINER TALK:

✔ Aim to perform your negative at a consistent pace. It's common to drop too quickly during the second half of the lowering phase, so be extra careful to go slowly from the time you reach a 90 degree angle at your elbows until you are in a dead hang.

✔ Though you will begin in an underhand false grip position, allow your hands to rotate outward as you descend.

Muscles Emphasized: Forearms, Lats, Pecs, Rear Deltoids, Rhomboids, Biceps, Abs

---

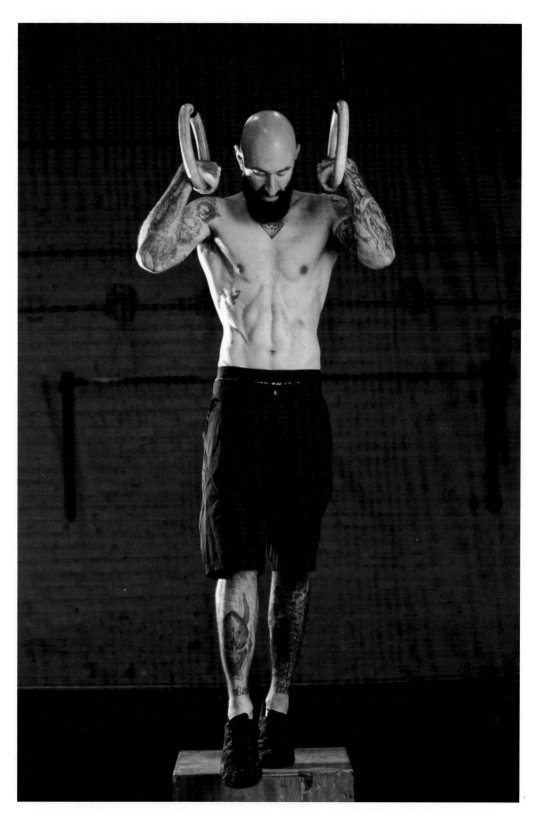

RINGS ASSISTED ARCHER SQUAT

1. Stand up straight with your feet in a very wide stance and toes angled outward to approximately 45 degrees, holding one ring in each hand at about chest height.

2. Shift your weight toward one side and begin squatting with that leg, while keeping your other leg straight. Descend until your hamstrings make contact with your calf, holding the rings for support as you extend your arms.

3. Pause briefly at the bottom before standing back up to the top position, gently pulling on the rings for assistance as needed, then repeat the movement on the opposite side.

TRAINER TALK:

✔ Be sure to keep the foot of your squatting leg flat on the ground the entire time. Allow the other foot to pivot into a toes-up position.

✔ Aim to rely on your arms only as needed, while doing the majority of the work with your legs.

**Muscles Emphasized:
Adductors, Quads,
Hamstrings, Glutes,
Calves, Low Back**

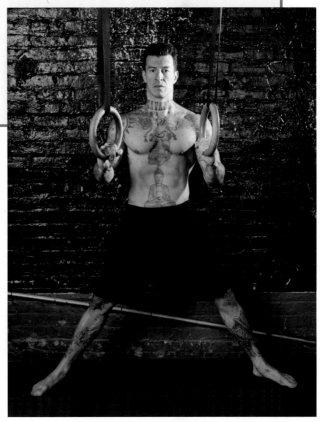

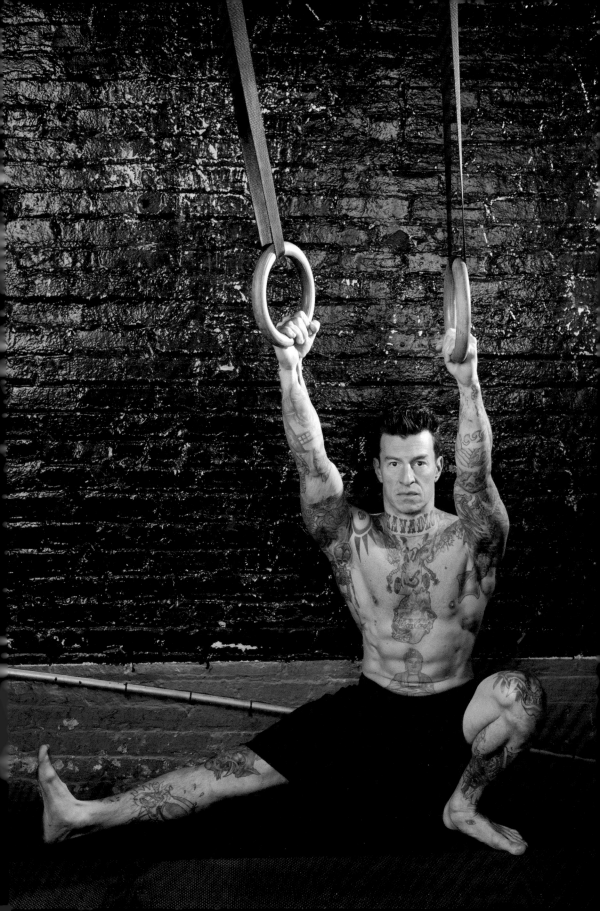

RINGS ASSISTED PISTOL SQUAT

1. Stand up straight with your feet approximately shoulder width apart, holding one ring in each hand at approximately chest height. Raise one leg in the air so it's straight out in front of you.

2. Extend your arms forward as you squat down from the hip, knee and ankle of your standing leg. Lower slowly until your hamstrings make contact with your calf. Keep the heel of your squatting leg flat on the ground the entire time.

3. Pause briefly at the bottom before standing back up to the top position, gently pulling on the rings for assistance only as needed. Repeat on the opposite side. Don't be thrown if one side is more difficult than the other. With practice the disparity should begin to even out.

TRAINER TALK:

✔ Be careful not to sit too far back during the lowering phase. Aim to travel purely up and down, though you may have to lean forward slightly in order to reach full depth.

✔ Don't be surprised if you feel your airborne leg working hard to keep from hitting the ground as you descend. It is a bit misleading to think of this as simply a one legged squat.

Muscles Emphasized: Quadriceps, Hamstrings, Glutes, Calves, Abs, Low Back, Hip Flexors

---

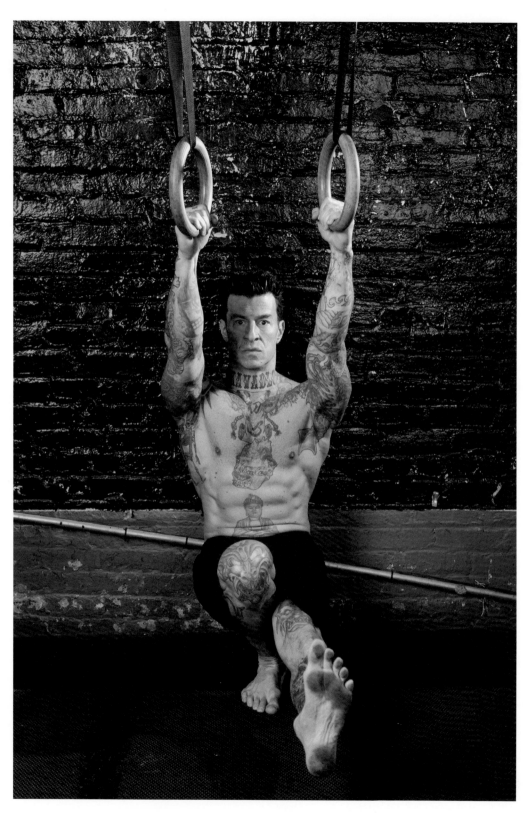

NEXT LEVEL STRENGTH

LEVEL 2—WEEKS 1 AND 2

✔ Repeat each of these workouts twice a week for the next two weeks, for a total of eight training sessions.

✔ You may perform Workout A and Workout B on consecutive days, but make sure you have at least 2 days in between repeating the same workout. For example, you may choose to do Workout A on Monday and Thursday, and Workout B on Tuesday and Friday.

✔ Begin each workout with the warm-up described earlier, then perform all exercises in sequence as written, resting for approximately 60-90 seconds between each set.

✔ Perform all reps with a controlled cadence and full range of motion.

✔ If you fail to complete the total necessary reps, you may add additional sets in order to get them finished.

✔ Do not move on until you can complete these workouts as written. If you cannot do so, then continue to repeat these workouts for as many weeks as necessary until you can.

WORKOUT A

Jump Through - 3 sets x 3 reps

L-sit - 3 sets x 5 second hold

Planche Lean -
3 sets x 5 second hold

Pike Press - 3 sets x 3 reps

Support Hold -
3 sets x 5 second hold

Inverted Hang -
3 sets x 5 second hold

Hanging Knee Raise -
3 sets x 10 reps

WORKOUT B

Pull-up - 3 sets x 3 reps

False Grip Flex Hang/Negative
Pull-up - 3 sets x 5 second hold +
5 second negative

Bodyweight Row - 3 sets x 10 reps

Rings Assisted Squat - 3 sets x 10 reps

Rings Assisted Archer Squat -
3 sets x 3 reps per leg

Rings Assisted Pistol Squat -
3 sets x 3 reps per leg

LEVEL 2—WEEKS 3 AND 4

✔ Repeat each of these workouts twice a week for the next two weeks, for a total of eight training sessions.

✔ You may perform Workout A and Workout B on consecutive days, but make sure you have at least 2 days in between repeating the same workout. For example, you may choose to do Workout A on Monday and Thursday, and Workout B on Tuesday and Friday.

✔ Begin each workout with the warm-up described earlier, then perform all exercises in sequence as written, resting for approximately 60-90 seconds between each set.

✔ Perform all reps with a controlled cadence and full range of motion.

✔ If you fail to complete the total necessary reps, you may add additional sets in order to get them finished.

✔ Do not move on until you can complete these workouts as written. If you cannot do so, then continue to repeat these workouts for as many weeks as necessary until you can.

WORKOUT A

Jump Through - 3 sets x 5 reps

L-sit - 3 sets x 10 second hold

Planche Lean -
3 sets x 10 second hold

Pike Press - 3 sets x 5 reps

Support Hold -
3 sets x 10 second hold

Inverted Hang -
3 sets x 10 second hold

Hanging Knee Raise -
3 sets x 10 reps

WORKOUT B

Pull-up - 3 sets x 5 reps

False Grip Flex Hang/Negative
Pull-up - 3 sets x 5 second hold +
10 second negative

Bodyweight Row - 3 sets x 10 reps

Rings Assisted Squat -
3 sets x 10 reps

Rings Assisted Archer Squat -
3 sets x 5 reps per leg

Rings Assisted Pistol Squat -
3 sets x 5 reps per leg

LEVEL 2—WEEKS 5 AND 6

✔ Repeat each of these workouts twice a week for the next two weeks, for a total of eight training sessions.

✔ You may perform Workout A and Workout B on consecutive days, but make sure you have at least 2 days in between repeating the same workout. For example, you may choose to do Workout A on Monday and Thursday, and Workout B on Tuesday and Friday.

✔ Begin each workout with the warm-up described earlier, then perform all exercises in sequence as written, resting for approximately 60-90 seconds between each set.

✔ Perform all reps with a controlled cadence and full range of motion.

✔ If you fail to complete the total necessary reps, you may add additional sets in order to get them finished.

✔ Do not move on until you can complete these workouts as written. If you cannot do so, then continue to repeat these workouts for as many weeks as necessary until you can.

WORKOUT A

Jump Through - 3 sets x 5 reps

L-sit - 3 sets x 15 second hold

Planche Lean -
3 sets x 15 second hold

Pike Press - 3 sets x 6 reps

Support Hold -
3 sets x 15 second hold

Inverted Hang -
3 sets x 15 second hold

Hanging Knee Raise -
3 sets x 10 reps

WORKOUT B

Pull-up - 3 sets x 6 reps

**False Grip Flex Hang/Negative
Pull-up** - 3 sets x 10 second hold +
10 second negative

Bodyweight Row - 3 sets x 10 reps

Rings Assisted Squat -
3 sets x 10 reps

Rings Assisted Archer Squat -
3 sets x 8 reps per leg

Rings Assisted Pistol Squat -
3 sets x 8 reps per leg

LEVEL 2—WEEKS 7 AND 8

✔ Repeat each of these workouts twice a week for the next two weeks, for a total of eight training sessions.

✔ You may perform Workout A and Workout B on consecutive days, but make sure you have at least 2 days in between repeating the same workout. For example, you may choose to do Workout A on Monday and Thursday, and Workout B on Tuesday and Friday.

✔ Begin each workout with the warm-up described earlier, then perform all exercises in sequence as written, resting for approximately 60-90 seconds between each set.

✔ Perform all reps with a controlled cadence and full range of motion.

✔ If you fail to complete the total necessary reps, you may add additional sets in order to get them finished.

✔ Do not move on until you can complete these workouts as written. If you cannot do so, then continue to repeat these workouts for as many weeks as necessary until you can.

✔ Once you can complete these workouts as written, take the Level 2 Test to see if you are ready to advance to the Next Level.

WORKOUT A

Jump Through - 3 sets x 6 reps

L-sit - 3 sets x 20 second hold

Planche Lean -
3 sets x 20 second hold

Pike Press - 3 sets x 8 reps

Support Hold -
3 sets x 20 second hold

Inverted Hang -
3 sets x 20 second hold

Hanging Knee Raise -
3 sets x 10 reps

WORKOUT B

Pull-up - 3 sets x 8 reps

False Grip Flex Hang/Negative
Pull-up - 3 sets x 15 second hold +
10 second negative

Bodyweight Row - 3 sets x 10 reps

Rings Assisted Squat -
3 sets x 10 reps

Rings Assisted Archer Squat -
3 sets x 10 reps per leg

Rings Assisted Pistol Squat -
3 sets x 10 reps per leg

LEVEL 2—TEST

If you can complete the following workout in sequence with less than 60 seconds between each exercise, then move on to Level 3 the following week. If you cannot complete the test as follows, repeat the last two weeks of training then test yourself again in two weeks' time.

You may choose to do the test in place of your third training day of week 8 or you may do it as the first day of the following week. Either way, give yourself two full days off from any formal strength training before and after attempting this test.

TAKE TWO FULL DAYS REST BEFORE THIS TEST

- ✔ Jump Through...8 reps
- ✔ L-sit ....30 second hold
- ✔ Planche Lean..30 second hold
- ✔ Pull-up...10 reps
- ✔ False Grip Flex Hang/ Negative Pull-up ....20 second hold + 10 second negative
- ✔ Pike Press ....10 reps
- ✔ Support Hold ....30 second hold
- ✔ Inverted Hang..30 second hold
- ✔ Rings Assisted Archer Squat ....15 reps per leg
- ✔ Rings Assisted Pistol Squat....................15 reps per leg

TAKE LEVEL 2 TEST

DID YOU PASS?

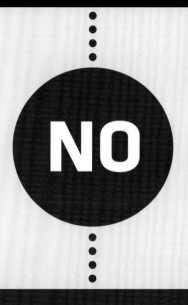

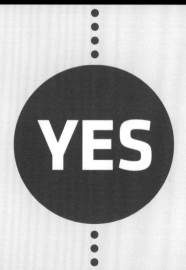

GO BACK TO LEVEL 2 WEEK 7

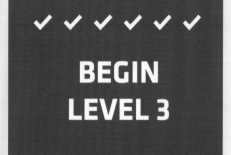

BEGIN LEVEL 3

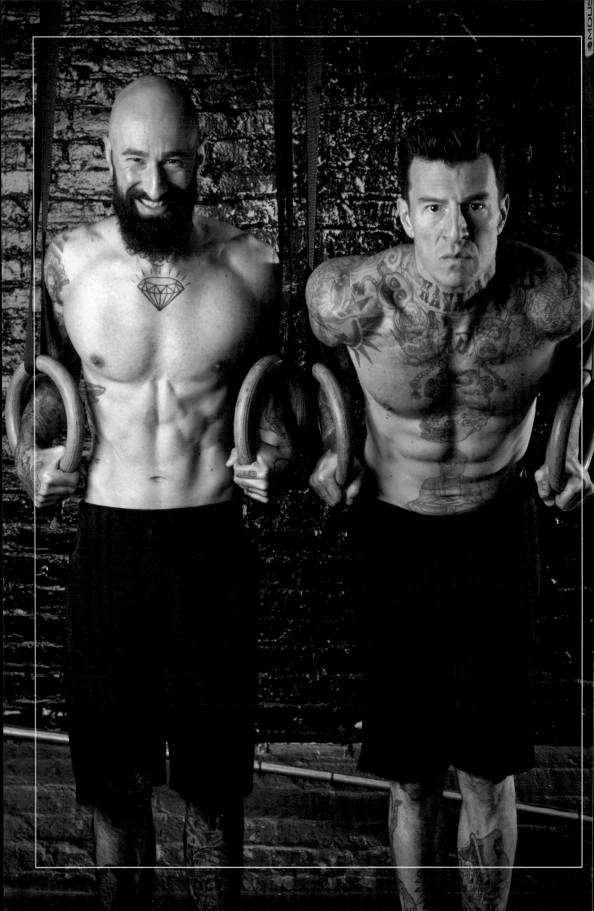

LEVEL 3

Indestructible

I f you've made it this far, you should be proud of your achievements. You have demonstrated a degree of dedication that is beyond what most people are willing to put forth when it comes to exercise. Now is the time to capitalize on your momentum and take things to the Next Level.

Stay on Level 3 for eight weeks, gradually increasing the number of reps performed on each exercise every two weeks as described in the programming ahead. You may notice that the increases in volume from workout to workout are a bit more gradual in this level. This is because more advanced exercises take longer to improve. You will see that not every exercise increases in reps or hold times from one workout to the next, though the overall workload will still increase gradually in preparation for the final test.

There are eight new exercises in level 3: Low Rings Push-up, Skin-the-Cat, L-sit to Tuck Planche, Elbow Lever, False Grip Pull-up, Dip, Single Ring Pistol Squat and Ring Assisted Shrimp Squat. You will also continue to use some of the exercises from previous levels.

For each new exercise, we've included a three-step description as well as "trainer talk" which provides further insight. Also included is a list of the muscles that are primarily emphasized. Be mindful, however, that all of these exercises employ the entire body to some degree.

After the exercises, there are charts containing specific program details including sets, reps and rest times. When you reach the end of this section there is a test to determine if you are ready to progress to the "Next" Next Level.

LOW RINGS PUSH-UP

1. Set your rings approximately 6-8 inches from the floor. Grab one ring in each hand from above, keeping your toes on the ground. Back your feet up so that you form a straight line from your heels to the back of your head. This will be your start position. You can try palms facing toward one another or palms facing down. Each position will place a slightly different emphasis on the muscles.

2. Keeping your whole body engaged, lower your chest toward your hands, allowing your shoulder blades to retract toward each other on the way down.

3. Carefully press yourself back to the start position, spreading your shoulder blades apart as your ascend. Be mindful not to let your shoulders shrug up toward your ears.

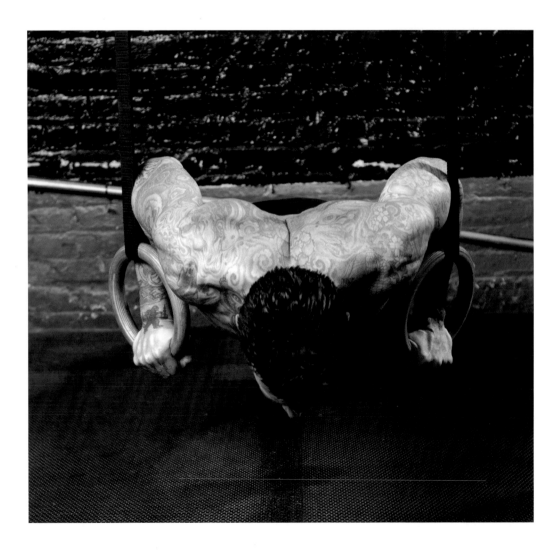

TRAINER TALK:

✔ If you aren't able to perform the exercise properly, you can try keeping your rings a bit higher for better leverage.

✔ You may find yourself swinging or shaking a bit on your first attempts. This is normal and should minimize with practice.

Muscles Emphasized: Pecs, Front Deltoids, Triceps, Abs

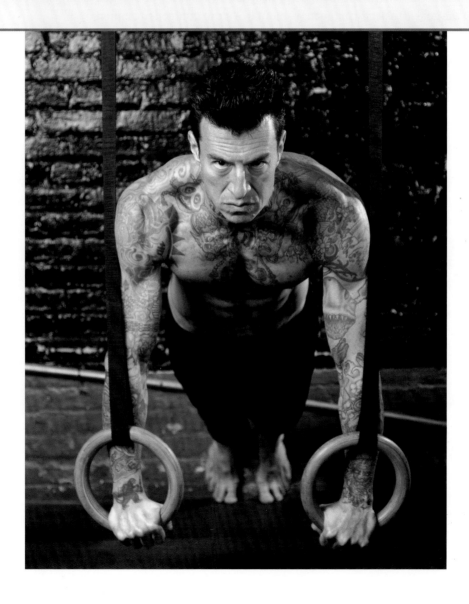

L-SIT TO TUCK PLANCHE

1. Begin in an L-sit, then tuck your knees toward your chest and bring your heels toward your butt.

2. Drag your hips back behind your hands, allowing your shoulders to drift forward as your hips rise until they are the same height as your shoulders. Your back should be slightly rounded with your shoulder blades spread apart.

3. Hold this position, then carefully return to the L-sit. That's one rep. You may use some momentum at first if you need to in order to get a taste of the tuck planche. Eventually the goal is to perform the movement in a slow, controlled fashion.

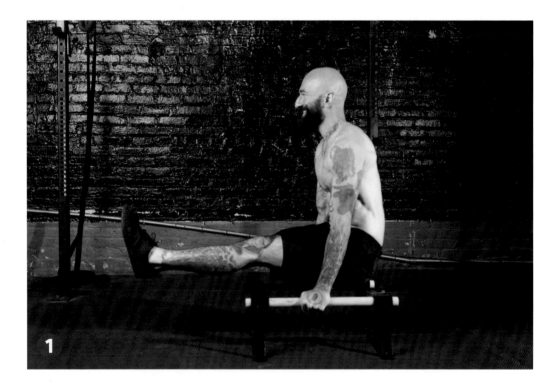

NEXT LEVEL STRENGTH

TRAINER TALK:

✔ As with the planche lean, it's important to flex your wrists in order to get the proper alignment. Your hands should wind up beneath your hips, not your shoulders.

✔ Think about actively squeezing your knees to your chest and lifting your heels toward your butt during the tuck planche part of the movement.

Muscles Emphasized: Abs, Pecs, Lats, Deltoids, Triceps, Hip Flexors, Quads

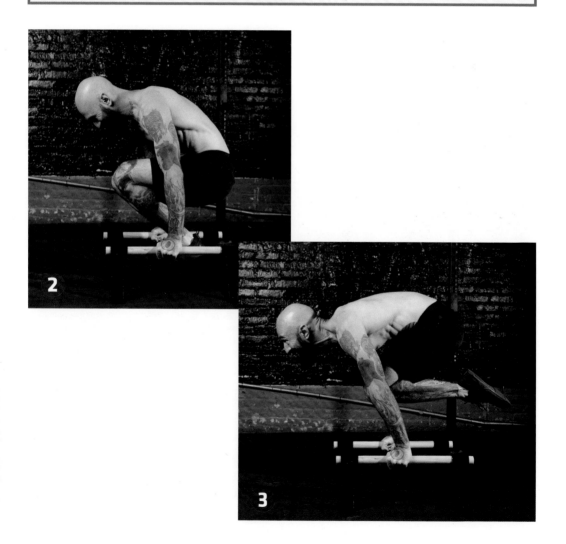

SKIN-THE-CAT

1. Hang below the rings in a standard grip, then bend your knees and lift them all the way toward your chest. When you can't get your knees any higher, rotate your body beneath the rings so your legs and feet pass behind them and onto the other side. Do your best to avoid bending your elbows. Pull from your lats with your arms straight. Think about driving the rings down toward your hips to help facilitate lifting your body higher.

2. Stay tucked until your body winds up behind the rings, then continue lowering yourself until your legs are fully extended with your arms positioned behind your back. Take your time in this position to make the most of the stretch. Folks with limited shoulder mobility will find this particularly important.

3. Return to the start position by tucking your knees toward your chest, bringing your heels toward your butt and threading yourself back around.

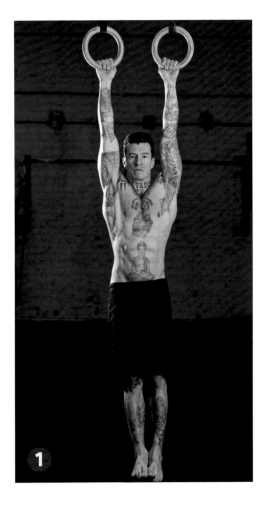
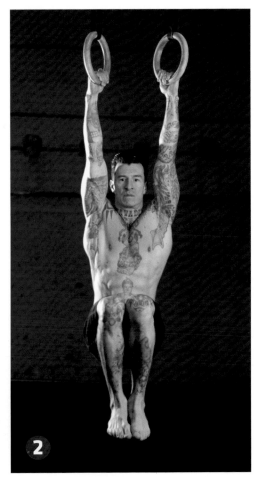

TRAINER TALK:

✔ In addition to the strength and mobility components, this exercise poses a serious spacial awareness challenge. You may start with your rings low to the ground so you can spot yourself with your feet and/or initiate the movement with a jump.

✔ To increase the difficulty, try performing this exercise with your legs straight.

Muscles Emphasized: Abs, Hip Flexors, Lats, Pecs, Deltoids

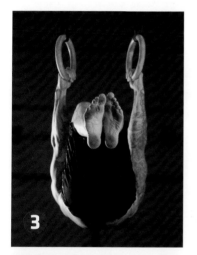

3

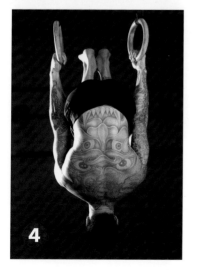

4

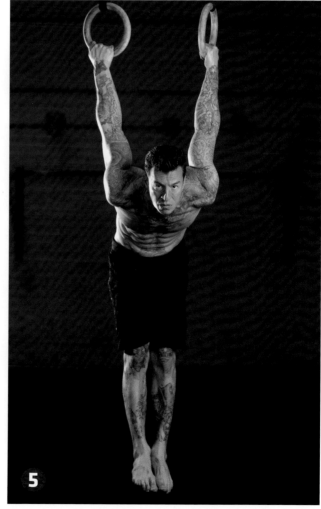

5

ELBOW LEVER

1. Grab your parallettes with one foot positioned in between your hands and your other foot outside of the bars.

2. Bend your elbows and lower yourself down until the elbow between your legs comes to rest against your hip on the same side.

3. Look forward and carefully shift your weight off of your feet until you are supported on just one elbow. Use your secondary arm for stability. If you aren't able to balance right away, keep one or both feet on the floor and practice putting as much weight as possible into your hands. Once you find the balance, keep your chest upright and fully extend both legs. Make sure to train both sides evenly.

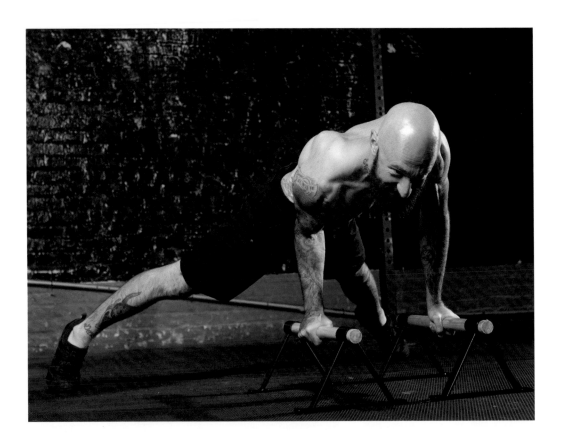

TRAINER TALK:

✔ The sensation of resting your hip against your elbow can feel uncomfortable at first, so don't be alarmed. This is normal.

✔ This position is typically easier to hold with your feet spread apart. To increase the difficulty, bring your legs closer to each other.

Muscles Emphasized: Abs, Front Deltoids, Pecs, Glutes, Low Back

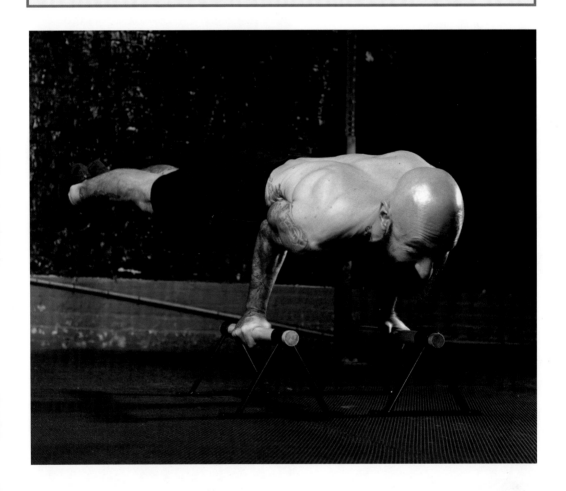

FALSE GRIP PULL-UP

1. Set the rings overhead and grasp one in each hand with an overhand false grip. It can help to stand on an elevated surface in order to set your grip before beginning your first rep.

2. Keep your abs braced and your legs straight as you pull your hands toward your shoulders while driving your elbows down to your hips. Keep your body as stable as possible. Do your best to avoid using any momentum.

3. When your chin is higher than your knuckles, carefully lower back to the bottom position.

TRAINER TALK:

✔ Focus on keeping your wrists flexed in order to maintain the false grip.

✔ Allow your hands to rotate as you pull. Most people will find that their hands naturally come to an underhand (or partially underhand) position at the top of the rep.

Muscles Emphasized: Forearms, Lats, Pecs, Rear Deltoids, Rhomboids, Biceps, Abs

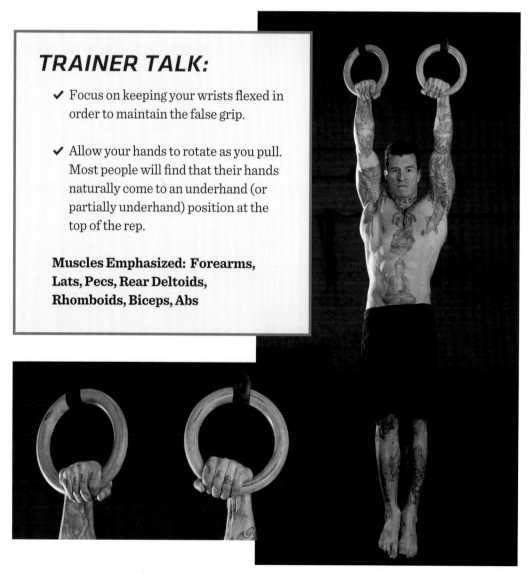

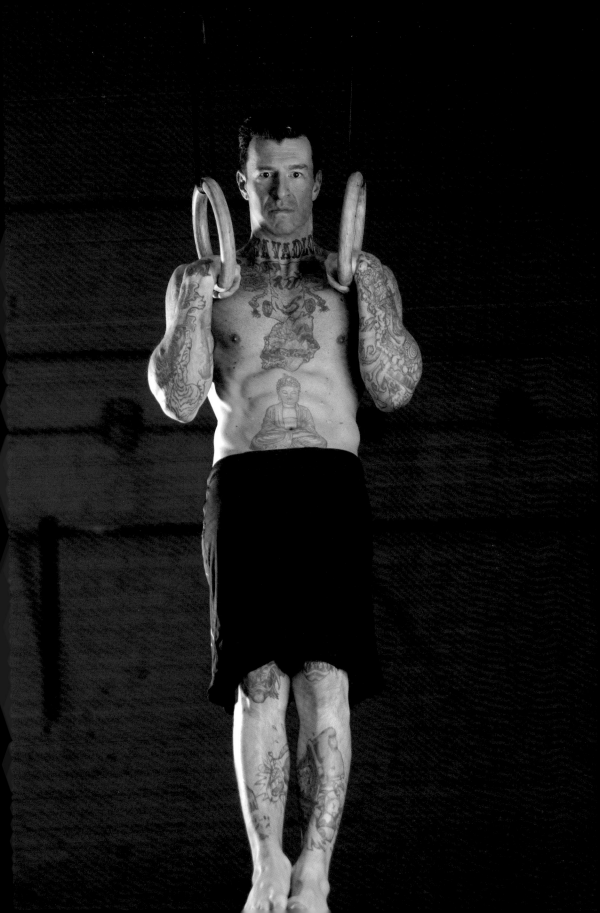

DIP

1. Begin in a support hold with your torso above the rings and your feet slightly in front of your body.

2. Bend your elbows and lean forward, lowering your chest toward your thumbs. You can keep your palms facing each other in a neutral grip or allow them to rotate to an overhand position at the bottom.

3. Press yourself back to the top position, keeping tension throughout your whole body. When your arms are fully extended, you may rotate your palms forward for an added challenge. Go slowly at first until you get comfortable with the movement pattern.

TRAINER TALK:

✔ If you are used to doing dips on bars or other stable surfaces, you may be surprised by the challenge presented by this variation.

✔ Keep your feet in front of your body. You may need to reach them further forward in the bottom position.

Muscles Emphasized: Pecs, Triceps, Front Deltoids

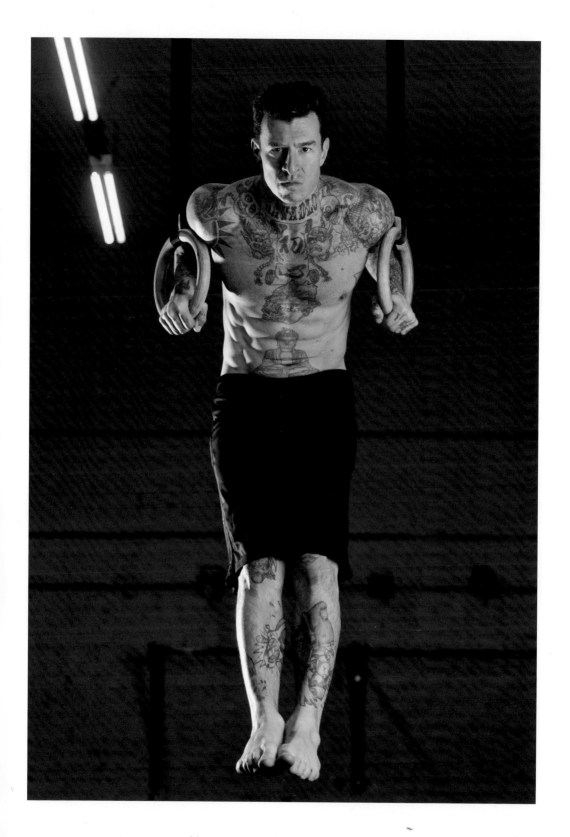

SINGLE RING PISTOL SQUAT

1. Stand up straight with your feet approximately shoulder width apart. Hold a single ring in your right hand at approximately chest height. Raise your right leg in the air in front of you and place your left hand behind your head. Keeping one hand behind your head offsets your center of gravity, rendering the exercise more difficult than when both arms are in front.

2. Extend your right arm forward as you squat down from the hip, knee and ankle of your left leg. Lower slowly until your hamstrings make contact with your calf. With only one arm assisting your squatting leg, the balance and stability demands are increased. Be sure to keep the heel flat on the ground the entire time.

3. Pause briefly at the bottom before standing back up to the top position, gently pulling on the ring for assistance as needed. Don't worry if one side is more difficult than the other. With practice the disparity should begin to even out.

TRAINER TALK:

✔ Be careful not to sit too far back during the lowering phase. Aim to travel purely up and down, though you may have to lean forward slightly in order to reach full depth.

✔ Don't be surprised if you feel your airborne leg working hard to keep from hitting the ground as you descend. It is a bit misleading to think of this as simply a one-legged squat.

Muscles Emphasized: Quadriceps, Hamstrings, Glutes, Calves, Abs, Low Back, Hip Flexors

---

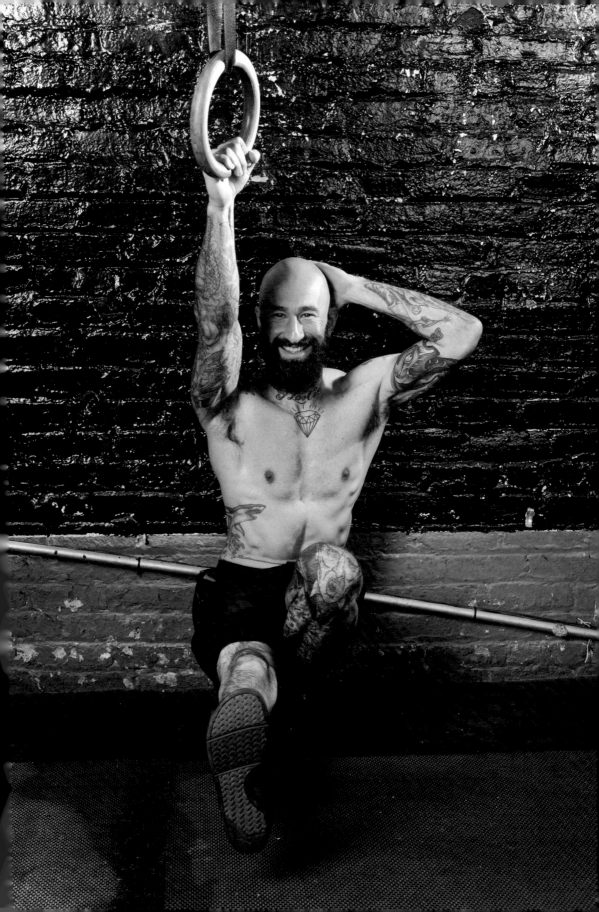

RING ASSISTED SHRIMP SQUAT

1. Stand up straight with your feet approximately shoulder width apart, holding a single ring in your right hand at approximately chest height. Bend your left leg and grab your left ankle behind your back, as though you were doing a standing quadriceps stretch.

2. Extend your right arm forward as you squat down from the hip, knee and ankle of your right leg. Keep your spine neutral and allow your torso to lean forward from your hips during the descent. Lower slowly until your knee gently touches down behind the heel of your squatting leg, keeping that heel flat on the ground the entire time.

3. Pause briefly at the bottom before standing back up to the top position, gently pulling on the ring for assistance only as needed.

TRAINER TALK:

✔ Don't be surprised if you feel a big stretch in your airborne leg. It is a bit misleading to think of this as simply a one-legged squat.

✔ If you are unable to perform this exercise, you can regress it by letting go of your airborne leg. Instead, use your other hand to hold a second ring for added stability.

Muscles Emphasized: Quadriceps, Hamstrings, Glutes, Calves, Abs, Low Back

---

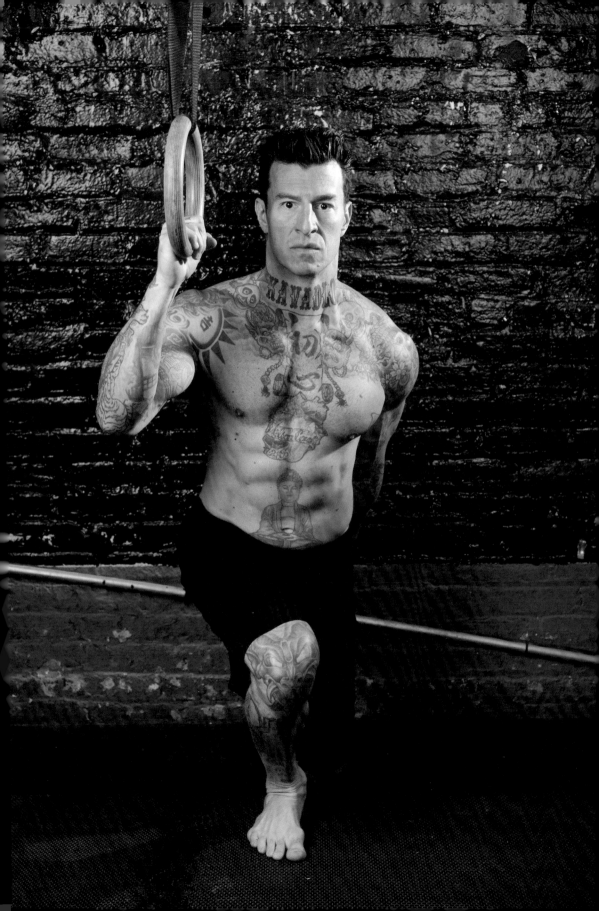

LEVEL 3—WEEKS 1 AND 2

✔ Repeat each of these workouts twice this week, for a total of four training sessions.

✔ You may perform Workout A and Workout B on consecutive days, but make sure you have at least 2 days in between repeating the same workout. For example, you may choose to do Workout A on Monday and Thursday, and Workout B on Tuesday and Friday.

✔ Begin each workout with the warm-up described earlier, then perform all exercises in sequence as written, resting for approximately 60-90 seconds between each set.

✔ Perform all reps with a controlled cadence and full range of motion.

✔ If you fail to complete the total necessary reps, you may add additional sets in order to get them finished.

✔ Do not move on until you can complete these workouts as written. If you cannot do so, then continue to repeat these workouts for as many weeks as necessary until you can.

WORKOUT A

L-sit to Tuck Planche
3 sets x 2 reps

Dip - 3 sets x 3 reps

Low Rings Push-up
3 sets x 5 reps

Pike Press - 3 sets x 5 reps

Elbow Lever
3 sets x 5 second hold per side

Inverted Hang
3 sets x 20 second hold

WORKOUT B

Skin-the-Cat - 3 sets x 1 rep

False Grip Pull-up - 3 sets x 3 reps

Pull-up - 3 sets x 5 reps

Bodyweight Row - 3 sets x 10 reps

Rings Archer Squat
3 sets x 10 reps

Single Ring Pistol Squat
3 sets x 5 reps per leg

Ring Assisted Shrimp Squat
3 sets x 5 reps per leg

LEVEL 3—WEEKS 3 AND 4

✔ Repeat each of these workouts twice this week, for a total of four training sessions.

✔ You may perform Workout A and Workout B on consecutive days, but make sure you have at least 2 days in between repeating the same workout. For example, you may choose to do Workout A on Monday and Thursday, and Workout B on Tuesday and Friday.

✔ Begin each workout with the warm-up described earlier, then perform all exercises in sequence as written, resting for approximately 60-90 seconds between each set.

✔ Perform all reps with a controlled cadence and full range of motion.

✔ If you fail to complete the total necessary reps, you may add additional sets in order to get them finished.

✔ Do not move on until you can complete these workouts as written. If you cannot do so, then continue to repeat these workouts for as many weeks as necessary until you can.

WORKOUT A

L-sit to Tuck Planche
3 sets x 3 reps

Dip - 3 sets x 5 reps

Low Rings Push-up
3 sets x 6 reps

Pike Press - 3 sets x 8 reps

Elbow Lever
3 sets x 10 second hold per side

Inverted Hang
3 sets x 30 second hold

WORKOUT B

Skin-the-Cat - 3 sets x 2 reps

False Grip Pull-up - 3 sets x 5 reps

Pull-up - 3 sets x 5 reps

Bodyweight Row - 3 sets x 10 reps

Rings Archer Squat
3 sets x 10 reps

Single Ring Pistol Squat
2 sets x 8 reps per leg

Ring Assisted Shrimp Squat
2 sets x 8 reps per leg

LEVEL 3—WEEKS 5 AND 6

✔ Repeat each of these workouts twice this week, for a total of four training sessions.

✔ You may perform Workout A and Workout B on consecutive days, but make sure you have at least 2 days in between repeating the same workout. For example, you may choose to do Workout A on Monday and Thursday, and Workout B on Tuesday and Friday.

✔ Begin each workout with the warm-up described earlier, then perform all exercises in sequence as written, resting for approximately 60-90 seconds between each set.

✔ Perform all reps with a controlled cadence and full range of motion.

✔ If you fail to complete the total necessary reps, you may add additional sets in order to get them finished.

✔ Do not move on until you can complete these workouts as written. If you cannot do so, then continue to repeat these workouts for as many weeks as necessary until you can.

WORKOUT A

L-sit to Tuck Planche -
3 sets x 4 reps

Dip - 3 sets x 6 reps

Low Rings Push-up -
3 sets x 8 reps

Pike Press - 3 sets x 10 reps

Elbow Lever -
3 sets x 15 second hold each side

Inverted Hang -
3 sets x 30 second hold

WORKOUT B

Skin-the-Cat - 3 sets x 3 reps

False Grip Pull-up - 3 sets x 5 reps

Pull-up - 3 sets x 6 reps

Bodyweight Row - 3 sets x 10 reps

Rings Archer Squat -
3 sets x 15 reps

Single Ring Pistol Squat -
2 sets x 10 reps per leg

Ring Assisted Shrimp Squat -
2 sets x 10 reps per leg

LEVEL 3—WEEKS 7 AND 8

✔ Repeat each of these workouts twice this week, for a total of four training sessions.

✔ You may perform Workout A and Workout B on consecutive days, but make sure you have at least 2 days in between repeating the same workout. For example, you may choose to do Workout A on Monday and Thursday, and Workout B on Tuesday and Friday.

✔ Begin each workout with the warm-up described earlier, then perform all exercises in sequence as written, resting for approximately 60-90 seconds between each set.

✔ Perform all reps with a controlled cadence and full range of motion.

✔ If you fail to complete the total necessary reps, you may add additional sets in order to get them finished.

✔ Do not move on until you can complete these workouts as written. If you cannot do so, then continue to repeat these workouts for as many weeks as necessary until you can.

✔ Once you can complete these workouts as written, take the Level 3 Test to see if you are ready to move ahead to the bonus exercises.

WORKOUT A

L-sit to Tuck Planche -
3 sets x 5 reps

Dip - 3 sets x 8 reps

Low Rings Push-up -
3 sets x 10 reps

Pike Press - 3 sets x 12 reps

Elbow Lever -
3 sets x 20 second hold per side

Inverted Hang -
3 sets x 30 second hold

WORKOUT B

Skin-the-Cat - 3 sets x 3 reps

False Grip Pull-up - 3 sets x 8 reps

Pull-up - 3 sets x 6 reps

Bodyweight Row - 3 sets x 10 reps

Rings Archer Squat -
3 sets x 15 reps

Single Ring Pistol Squat -
2 sets x 12 reps per leg

Ring Assisted Shrimp Squat -
2 sets x 12 reps per leg

LEVEL 3–TEST

The following test consists of all the new exercises from this level. Complete the test in sequence with less than 60 seconds between each exercise, and you have officially achieved Next Level Strength. Congratulations!

If you cannot complete the test as follows, repeat the last two weeks of training then test yourself again in two weeks' time.

You may choose to do the test in place of your third training day of week 8 or you may do it as the first day of the following week. Either way, give yourself two full days off from any formal strength training before and after attempting this test.

TAKE *TWO FULL DAYS REST* BEFORE THIS TEST

- ✔ L-sit to Tuck Planche ....5 reps
- ✔ Dip ....10 reps
- ✔ Low Rings Push-up....................................20 reps
- ✔ Elbow Lever ....30 second hold per side
- ✔ Skin-the-Cat ....5 reps
- ✔ False Grip Pull-up....................................10 reps
- ✔ Single Ring Pistol Squat..........................15 reps per leg
- ✔ Ring Assisted Shrimp Squat ....15 reps per leg

TAKE LEVEL 3 TEST

DID YOU PASS?

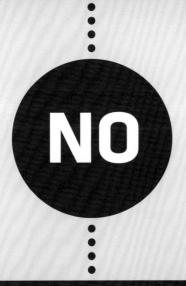

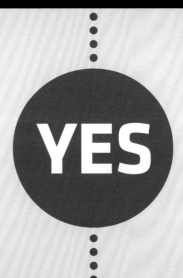

GO BACK TO LEVEL 3 WEEK 7

HELLYEAH! WE'RE WORKING OUT!

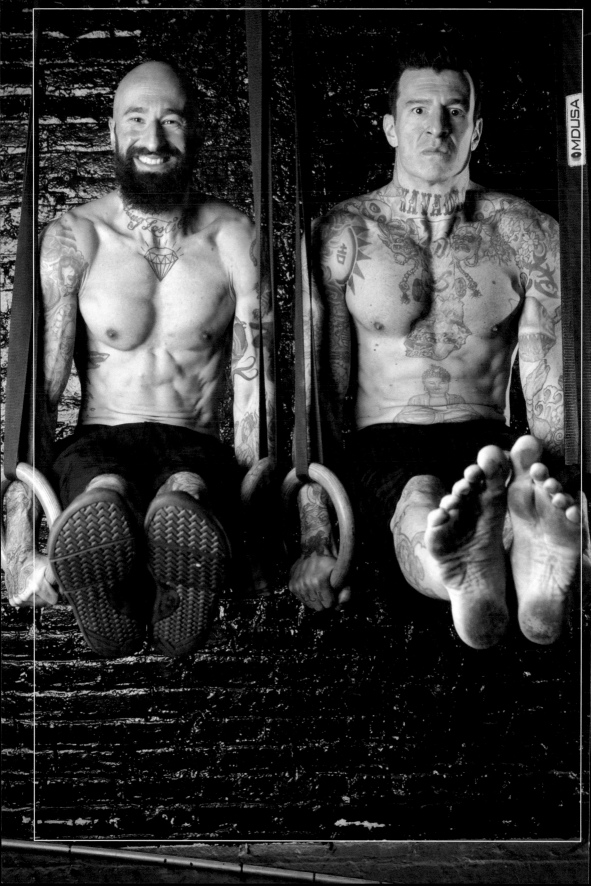

The "Next" Next Level

Now that you have built Next Level Strength, you are ready to tackle the following eight new exercises: Parallettes Handstand, Parallettes Handstand Push-up, Rings L-sit, V-sit, Muscle-up, Back Lever, Front Lever and One-Arm Elbow Lever. These are all high-level pursuits, so take your time and try not to get discouraged if some of them seem impossible at first. We assure you the work you've done so far has not been in vain, but these exercises may make you feel like a beginner all over again.

For each new exercise, we've included a three-step description as well as "trainer talk" which provides further insight. Also included is a list of the muscles that are primarily emphasized. Be mindful, however, that all of these exercises employ the entire body to some degree.

There is no timeline for learning these exercises, as it can take months or even years to conquer these behemoths. You can't force fitness, so be patient and enjoy the ride. See the "Programming Your Workouts" section in Part II for guidance on how to incorporate these exercises into your own custom training plan.

PARALLETTES HANDSTAND

1. Place your parallettes near a wall. Grip them so your hands are positioned approximately 6-8 inches from the wall.

2. With your elbows fully locked, kick your legs into the air until your heels come to rest against the wall. If you're having trouble kicking up, it can help to think about getting your hips over your hands rather than focusing on your legs. Either way, don't let your elbows bend.

3. Hold this position, then come down as gently as possible. With continued practice you will learn to rely less on the wall until you are able to perform a freestanding handstand.

TRAINER TALK:

✔ Many people will find it helpful to look in between their hands while performing this hold, though others will prefer to keep their head in a neutral position.

✔ The farther your bars are from the floor, the harder you will need to kick in order to get into position.

Muscles Emphasized: Deltoids, Traps, Pecs, Triceps

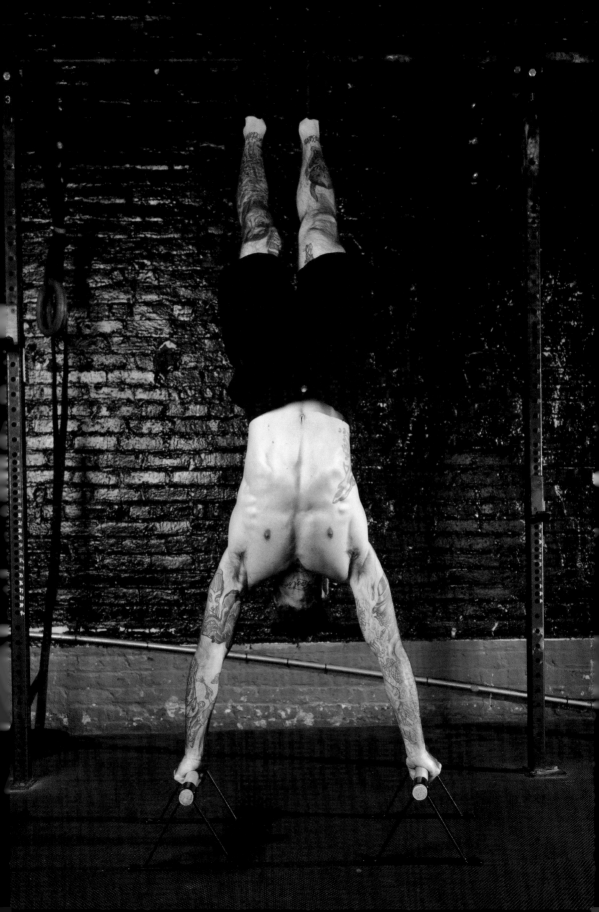

PARALLETTES HANDSTAND PUSH-UP

1. Begin in the handstand position.

2. Look in front of your hands. Bend your arms and carefully lower your head toward the ground. Do not allow your elbows to flare out to the sides.

3. Pause briefly before your head touches the ground, then press yourself back to the top. Make sure to keep your hips directly above your shoulders the whole time. You may need to arch your back a bit in order to facilitate the full range of motion, however, aim to keep any arching to a minimum.

TRAINER TALK:

✔ If you aren't able to lower yourself all the way down, you can start with a partial range of motion.

✔ With continued practice you can gradually rely less on the wall until you are able to perform a freestanding handstand push-up.

Muscles Emphasized: Deltoids, Traps, Pecs, Triceps, Abs

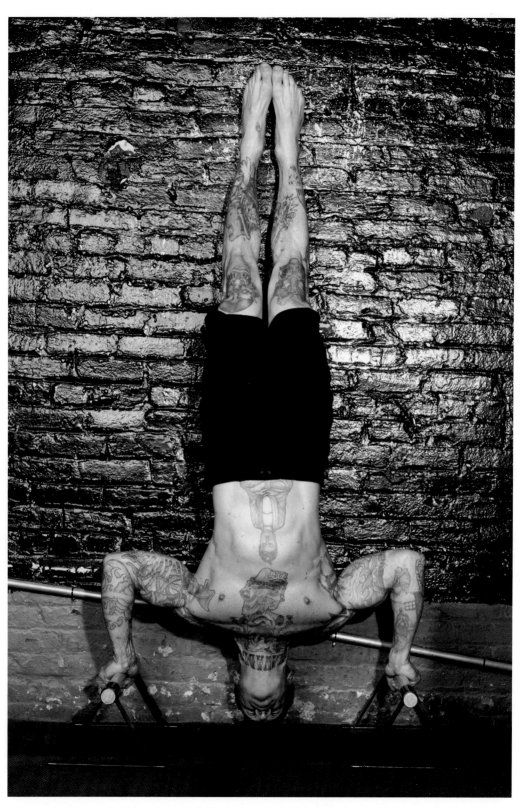

RINGS L-SIT

1. Begin in a support hold above the rings.

2. Keep your arms locked as you carefully raise your legs straight out in front of your body, forming a shape like a capital letter "L". Press down into the rings, point your elbow pits forward and allow your upper back to round slightly so that you can spread your shoulder blades apart, being mindful not to let your shoulders shrug up toward your ears.

3. You may point or flex your toes. Either way make sure your feet remain engaged. You may find yourself swinging or shaking a bit on your first attempts. This is normal and should minimize with practice.

TRAINER TALK:

✔ For an added challenge, try rotating your palms forward.

Muscles Emphasized:
Abs, Pecs, Triceps,
Lats, Deltoids,
Hip Flexors, Quads

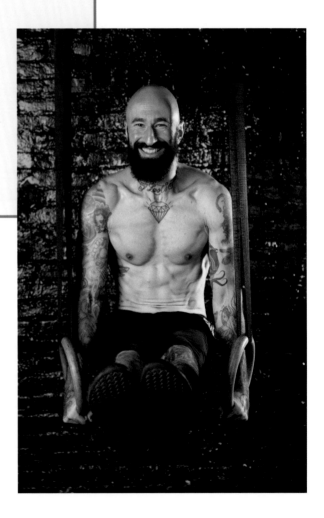

V-SIT

1. Grab your parallettes with your torso upright and your shoulders and hips directly above your hands. Your feet will be flat on the floor with your knees bent.

2. Press down into the handles, point your elbow pits forward and allow your upper back to round slightly so that you can spread your shoulder blades apart, being mindful not to let your shoulders shrug up toward your ears.

3. Lift your feet off the floor, extending your legs up and away from your body. You will need to lean your torso back and hips forward in order to raise your legs higher. The shape of your body will resemble a capital letter "V". You may point or flex your toes. Either way make sure your feet remain engaged. You may find yourself swinging or shaking a bit on your first attempts. This is normal and should minimize with practice.

TRAINER TALK:

✔ Focus on getting your hips farther in front of your hands in order to facilitate lifting your legs higher.

✔ If you aren't able to perform the exercise with both legs fully extended, you can try bending one or both knees.

Muscles Emphasized: Abs, Pecs, Triceps, Lats, Deltoids, Hip Flexors, Quads

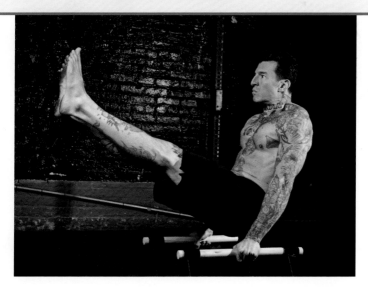

MUSCLE-UP

1. Set the rings overhead and grasp one in each hand using an overhand false grip. It can help to stand on an elevated surface in order to set your grip before beginning your first rep.

2. Reach your legs forward and begin pulling your hands toward your armpits while driving your elbows down and back. Keep your body as stable as possible and do your best to avoid using momentum.

3. Once the rings are below your shoulders, push your chest and shoulders in front of your hands so your knuckles wind up facing the ground. Then extend your arms to complete the rep. Reverse the movement pattern to come back to the start position.

TRAINER TALK:

✔ Allow the rings to rotate as you move through the transition phase.

✔ If you are struggling with this exercise, it can help to practice a "negative muscle-up" by slowly lowering yourself down through the transition phase from the support hold, similarly to how you practiced negative pull-ups in Level 1.

Muscles Emphasized:
Forearms, Lats, Pecs, Deltoids,
Rhomboids, Biceps, Triceps, Abs

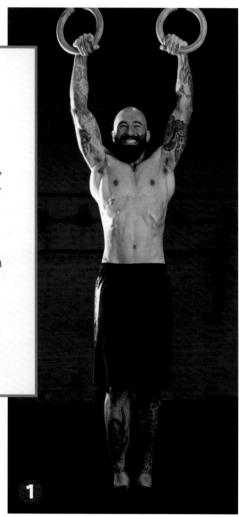

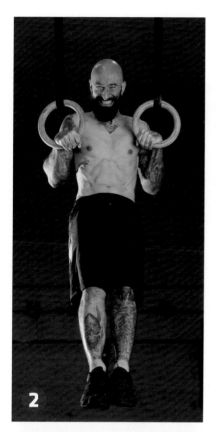

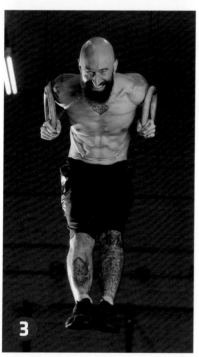

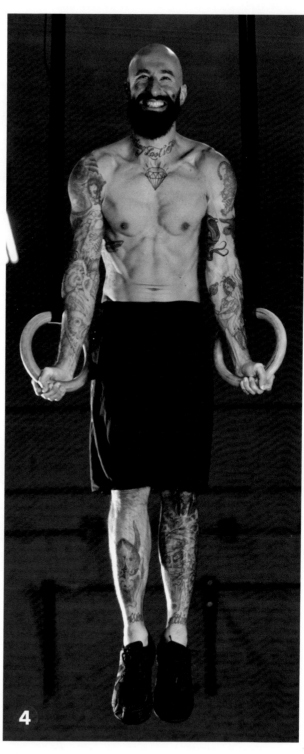

BACK LEVER

1. Begin in an inverted hang, looking toward the floor.

2. Carefully start lowering your body toward a face-down horizontal position. Pitch your chest forward as you descend so your hands wind up behind your lower back. Shift your gaze forward as you get closer to parallel to the ground.

3. Squeeze your arms close to your sides as you continue lowering your body until you are completely horizontal. Engage your abdominals in order to minimize any arching of your back. Aim to form as straight of a line as possible. You can experiment with different hand positions. Most people will find that palms facing upward is less difficult than palms facing the ground.

TRAINER TALK:

✔ If you are unable to perform the full movement with both legs fully extended, you can regress the exercise by bending one or both knees and tucking your leg(s) toward your chest.

✔ Once you can hold a full back lever, you can try lifting into position from the bottom of a skin-the-cat, rather than lowering yourself down from an inverted hang.

Muscles Emphasized: Lats, Biceps, Pecs, Deltoids, Rhomboids, Low Back, Glutes, Abs

---

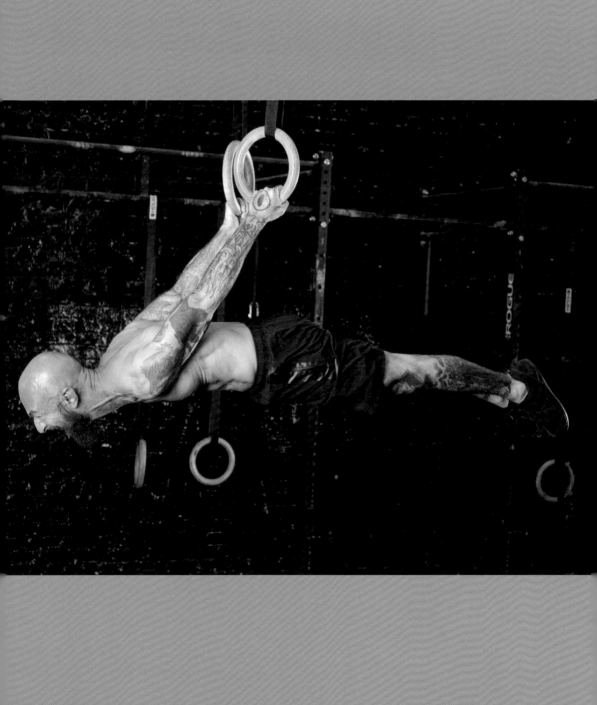

FRONT LEVER

1. Begin in an inverted hang, looking toward your toes.

2. Carefully start lowering your body into a face-up horizontal position, while simultaneously leaning back from your upper body so the rings wind up above your hips. Make sure your arms remain straight.

3. Squeeze your arms close to your sides as you continue lowering your body until you are completely horizontal. Engage your abs in order to minimize any bend at the hips. Aim to form as straight of a line as possible.

TRAINER TALK:

✔ If you are unable to perform the full movement with both legs fully extended, regress the exercise by bending one or both knees and tucking your leg(s) toward your chest.

✔ Once you can hold a full front lever, you can try lifting into position from a standard hang, rather than lowering yourself down from an inverted hang.

Muscles Emphasized: Lats, Pecs, Deltoids, Abs, Glutes, Triceps

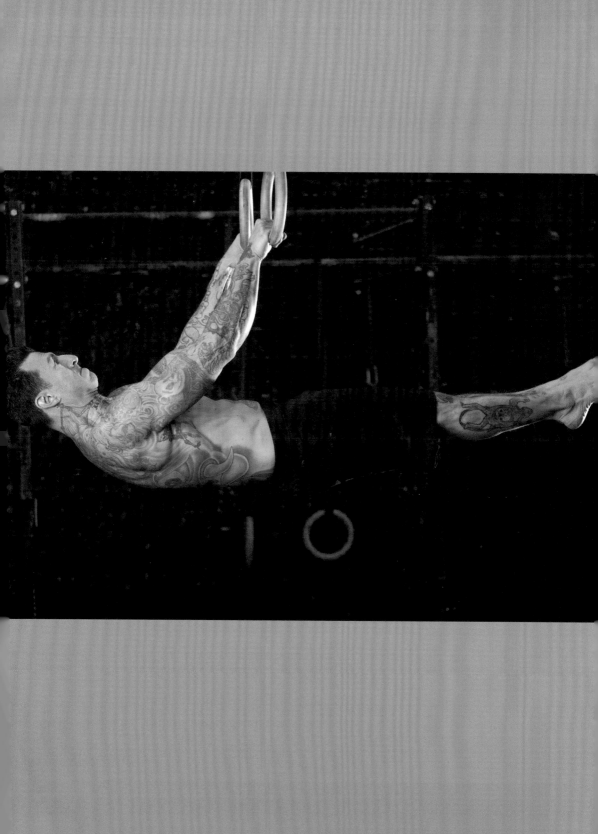

ONE-ARM ELBOW LEVER

1. Begin in the standard elbow lever position.

2. Slowly shift your weight toward the hand that is beneath your hip. Reach your free arm away from your body to help balance, gradually taking weight away from it.

3. With enough practice, you will eventually be able to remove your secondary hand entirely. Make sure to practice on both sides in order to keep things even.

TRAINER TALK:

✔ When starting out, it's generally best to keep your feet spread apart. Once you can balance on one hand, try bringing your legs closer together to make it more difficult.

✔ As you get closer to the full expression of the exercise, try practicing with your secondary arm farther from your body to help shift more weight to your primary arm. You can also practice with your assisting hand directly on the ground.

Muscles Emphasized: Abs, Front Deltoids, Pecs, Glutes, Low Back

---

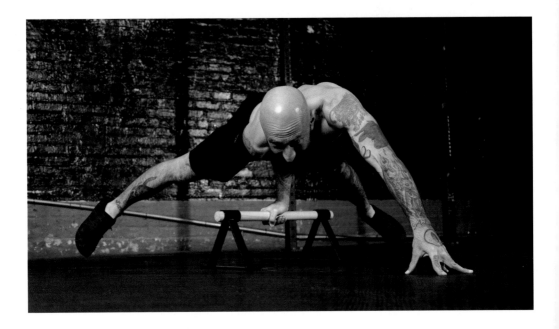

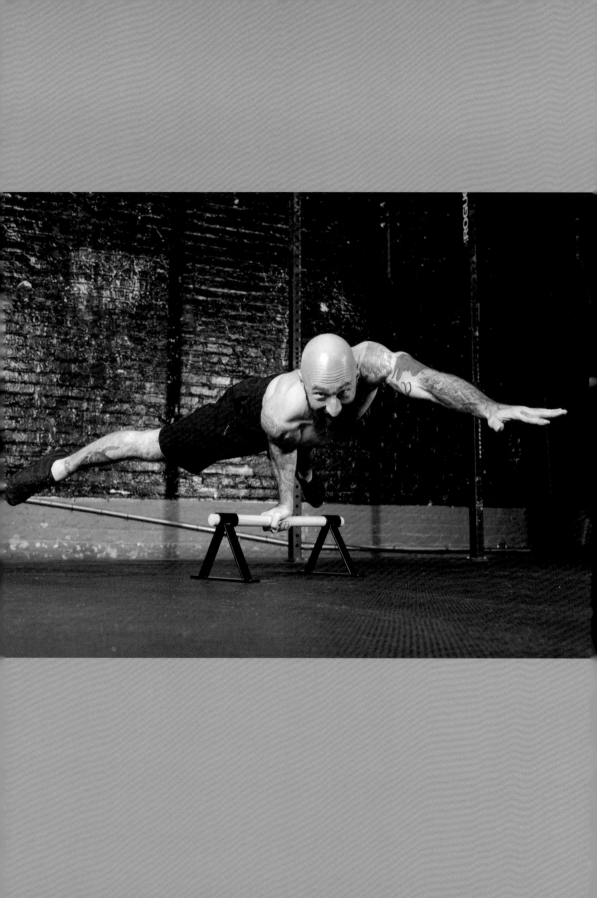

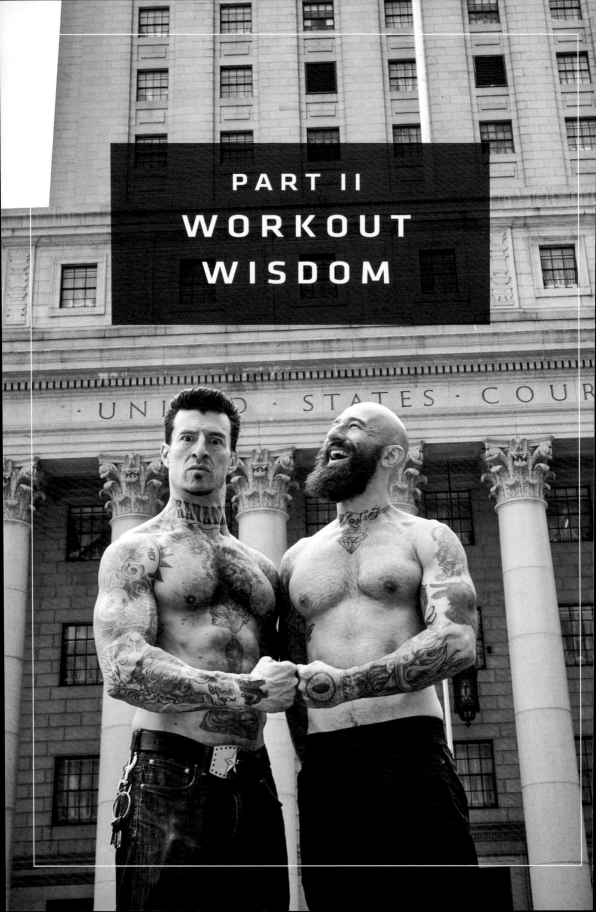

PART II
WORKOUT
WISDOM

Moving Ahead with the Beginner's Mind

I t has been said that, "In the beginner's mind there are many possibilities, but in the expert's mind there are few." This means that no matter how much knowledge you acquire, it's still in your best interest to stay receptive to new ideas. We encourage you to approach fitness with this mindset. Regardless of your previous experience, what lies ahead may be different from what you expect.

If you've completed the Next Level Strength program, you have accomplished a huge achievement, but your journey does not need to end there. After you finish the program, it's time for you to take the reins. We want to empower you to design your own training plan. We will teach you how.

In "Programming Your Workouts" we'll show you how you can create training templates to take with you for the rest of your life. This information will prove invaluable throughout your practice.

"Ask Al" shares answers to some of the most frequently asked questions about the Next Level Strength program, training, health and life. You will enjoy Al's insights on a wide variety of topics from the esoteric to the existential.

To truly take it to the Next Level, there is much to consider beyond your training.

"Danny's Dos and Don'ts" will give you the real deal on commitment, sacrifice and recovery, not to mention some of the most detailed nutritional guidance we've ever put into print.

Embrace the beginner's mind. Let's move ahead!

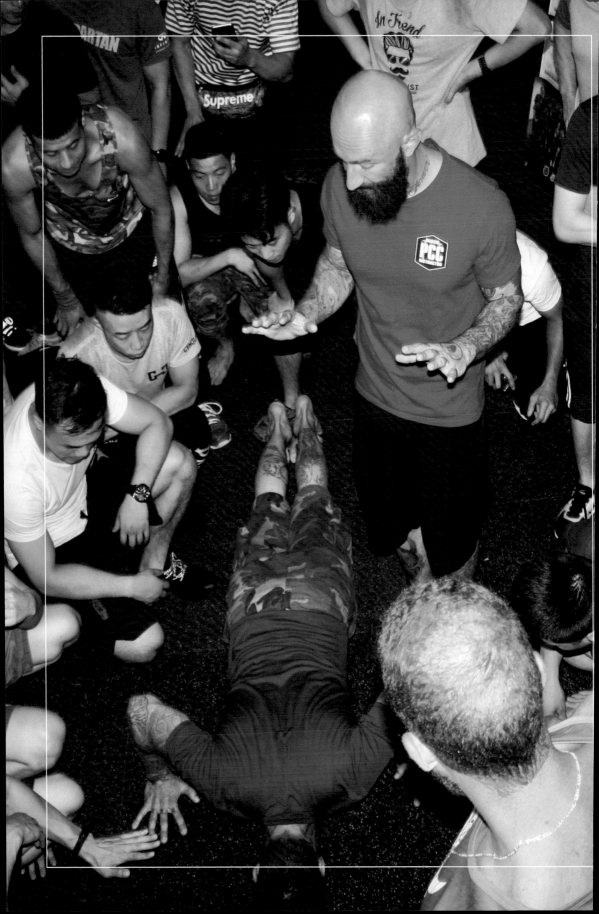

Programming Your Workouts

L ike the old saying goes, "Give a person a fish and they'll eat one meal but teach that person to fish and they'll eat for a lifetime."

When designing your own personalized exercise program, there are many variables to consider, including exercise selection, set/rep schemes, rest times and more. Programming your own workout may seem daunting, but when you think about it, who knows you better than you do? And who better to design your workout than you?

In fact, if you've completed the Next Level Strength program, you've already been peripherally learning about program design simply by following the workouts we've prescribed. Now it's just a matter of dissecting the details and distilling them down to universally applicable concepts.

We've taught these tenets to trainers, coaches and other fitness professionals all over the world. Now we're sharing them with you.

Let's go fishing!

EXERCISE SELECTION

The Next Level Strength program was designed with strength and muscle building as the primary goals, but regardless of your goal, progress only happens when you work near the fringes of your capabilities. Straddling the line between your current competencies and things that are just outside your reach is what causes adaptation. Just as you won't achieve anything without pushing yourself, you also won't achieve much if you push too hard, too soon.

With that in mind, you need to be sure that you're choosing appropriate exercises for yourself and your goal. When going for endurance, you'll want to do more reps of relatively easy exercises in fewer sets. If you're pursuing pure strength, you'll want to do the opposite: harder moves, fewer reps and lots of rest in between. In this case, you should also spread your reps out over more sets to keep from running out of energy too quickly.

Different people will respond differently, but for most individuals, hypertrophy (muscle growth) happens somewhere between those two ends of the spectrum. However, there are many ways to split the difference. Obviously, there is an overlap between these goals and none of them can be completely isolated.

Use this chart for general reference:

Goal	Rep Range*	Set Range	Rest Between Sets
Strength	1-6	5-10	3-5 minutes
Hypertrophy	6-25	3-5	1-3 minutes
Endurance	25+	2-3	<60 seconds

*For isometric holds, multiply this number by 3 and hold for that many seconds

To be perfectly clear, if you're planning an endurance workout, you have to pick exercises that you can actually do for lots of reps with clean form. If you're trying to build strength, you should pick something very challenging in the lower rep range. If you've made it through Next Level Strength and you want to keep getting stronger, doing five sets of five bodyweight rows, for example, will not get you very far. Five sets of five muscle-ups, however, is a different story. Just remember to keep your expectations reasonable. If you're still struggling to hold an elbow lever with both arms, trying the one-arm version is unlikely to be a fruitful pursuit.

Also bear in mind that as you build strength and muscle, exercises that were once very difficult can become more comfortable. In the beginning, a push-up with the rings set at waist height might be enough to fatigue you in 10 reps, making it primarily a strength and mass building move. After a couple of months of consistent training, however, your strength will have increased and you may find that exercise better suited to an endurance workout requiring a greater number of repetitions. Again, there will always be some overlap in training for strength, hypertrophy and/or endurance.

FREQUENCY AND INTENSITY

Regardless of the specific exercises you choose to focus on, frequency and intensity are the two most important variables that you can modify to suit your goals.

Frequency refers to how often you train; intensity is how much effort you expend. Though the specifics will change as you progress, these variables will remain consistent relative to your fitness level. So no matter how strong you get, you'll always need to push yourself hard if you wish to continue progressing. But you also need adequate rest. Finding the sweet spot can be an elusive equation.

The ratio between frequency and intensity is the key to determining how much rest you will need between workouts, as well as between exercises. It applies to both your overall training schedule as well as any given exercise in your program. As one goes up, the other must go down. This means you will need more rest after a very intense workout before your next training session. It also means that you should not expect to perform as many reps of a more difficult exercise as you would a less difficult one. Furthermore, you will need a longer rest period after performing a very intense exercise before you will be able to do your next set. So if you only train the most difficult moves, you will burn yourself out quickly unless you keep your training volume relatively low. Conversely, when you focus on less difficult progressions, you'll need to increase your frequency in order to effect change.

PERIODIZATION

If you've spent the last several weeks or months training predominantly for strength, it can be helpful to switch your program to a more endurance or hypertrophy based template. This is beneficial for several reasons:

✔ Your nervous system gets a break from constantly working near peak intensity.

✔ It may prevent boredom and other mental plateaus.

✔ Your tendons, ligaments and other connective tissue get additional time to adapt.

✔ You may make better strength gains down the line.

You read that right: Training for endurance can set you up to make better strength gains down the line. You see, the more you increase your work capacity through muscular endurance training, the better prepared you will be to handle a higher training volume, which can ultimately allow you to build more strength and muscle. Though at first glance it may seem contrary to what we said previously, strength and endurance are not necessarily on opposite sides of the spectrum.

If you look closely at how the Next Level Strength program progresses, you will notice that each level gradually builds in training volume. When a level is completed, the volume at the start of the following level drops considerably in order to account for the increased difficulty of the exercises. Then it gradually builds up again. This is periodization in action.

EXERCISE SEQUENCING

We like to begin each session with a general warm-up. After the warm-up, we suggest you perform one or two medium-intensity exercises. At this point, while still early in your workout, it's time for the most difficult or demanding exercises. These can be either the toughest moves, the ones that incorporate the largest muscles or the big, compound movements with the highest energy expenditure. We don't recommend doing more than two or three of your most difficult exercises per body part in a single workout.

Employing this method allows you to give your best effort to the most challenging exercises after you're warmed up, but while you're still fresh. Once you've completed the most demanding exercises, you should move onto less intense ones for the remainder of your workout. Because of the amount of energy required earlier on, these later exercises, though seemingly less difficult, are unlikely to feel that way.

Moreover, you can choose to shift your emphasis from body part to body part with each exercise. This practice is based on the principle of "active recovery." While the muscles that are primarily emphasized during the first exercise recover, you can target different ones before moving ahead. Another method is to exhaust one muscle group entirely before switching your emphasis to the next area.

There are many ways to approach exercise sequencing and folks have gotten results with almost all of them, provided they put in the work. At the end of the day, you may find that the intensity of your effort will play the greatest role in your progress, regardless of how you sequence your exercises.

LEVERAGE

When working toward advanced moves, it helps to understand how to scale them to your capabilities. Everyone knows that a push-up on your knees is less difficult than one performed on your toes—but why is this so? The answer is leverage. The longer you make your body, the farther your arms wind up from your fulcrum point, creating more resistance.

Though the push-up might be the most obvious way to conceptualize this idea, it can be applied to many advanced calisthenics moves like the back lever and front lever, both of which can be first approached with the legs in a tucked position. From there you can progress to a single leg tuck and then a straddle leg position before finally performing either move with both legs together and fully extended. The more you extend your leg(s) the harder these moves become.

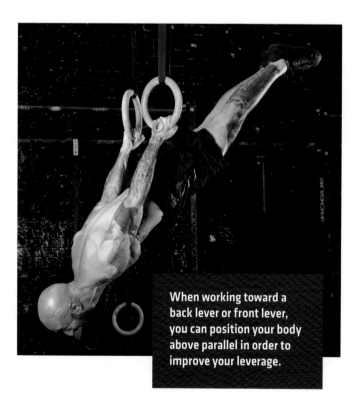

When working toward a back lever or front lever, you can position your body above parallel in order to improve your leverage.

Another way that this concept can be applied is by changing the angle of your entire body rather than just the position of your legs. When working toward a back lever or front lever, for example, you can position your body above parallel in order to improve your leverage. The closer you are to vertical, the easier the exercise becomes. This can allow you to get a feel for the full expression of the exercise without having to overcome as much resistance.

This concept is also why a push-up with your rings set high is less difficult than one with the rings close to the ground. The higher up your hands are, the closer your body gets to being vertical, once again rendering the exercise less difficult.

When you utilize leverage to alter your resistance, the scalability of any given exercise becomes virtually limitless. The height of your rings can be subtly adjusted to an infinite degree, as can the position of your legs. The smallest changes can sometimes make a big difference in your training.

RANGE OF MOTION

If you're not able to do a pull-up yet, but have enough grip strength to hang from the rings, one of the first things to work on is the flex hang and negative pull-up. By simply holding the top position, then lowering down slowly, you're able to build strength and get a feel for the movement pattern without having to concern yourself with the pulling phase. You are only practicing half of the movement. This is one example of using a limited range of motion to regress an exercise.

Another example would be for individuals who are unable to go all the way down on a squat. In this instance they could start out with a half squat, over time working toward increasing their mobility until they can perform a full range of motion with their hamstrings touching their calves in the bottom position.

The concept can also be used to make an exercise more difficult instead. After all, why is a muscle-up so much more work than a pull-up? It might have something to do with the fact that you are moving your body through a much greater range of motion. Rather than stopping when your chin is above your hands, the muscle-up continues until your entire upper body is above the rings in a support hold.

Decreasing your range of motion will usually make an exercise less difficult, while increasing your range of motion will almost always increase the difficulty.

SELF ASSISTANCE

Just like with pull-ups, if you haven't gotten your first muscle-up yet, it can help to practice negatives. In either case, it can also be helpful to give yourself some assistance by pushing off the ground with your feet as needed. The notion of self assistance can be applied to most calisthenics exercises.

The reason we suggest performing squats (even advanced squats like pistols and shrimps) while holding onto rings is so that you can provide yourself with just enough assistance to perform the repetition with good form, but not so much as to render the exercise less effective.

Just as when you're spotted by a partner, it's best when the amount of assistance is minimal. There is a delicate art to assisting anybody, even yourself. Once you understand this, you can always find a way to scale a difficult exercise.

PROGRESS AND SPECIFICITY

As trainers, one of the most common questions we get asked is, "What's the best way to nail your first muscle-up (or front lever, handstand, etc.)?"

Though the people asking these questions are typically hoping to discover a secret, trick, hack or shortcut, our answer is always to do the work.

There is a concept in exercise science that's referred to as the "specificity principle." It's basically a fancy way of saying that you get better at the things which you consistently practice. As you continue to refine exercises like the L-sit or muscle-up, for example, you will no longer shake as much as you did in the beginning. The moves become smoother and feel more comfortable the more that you do them. While this is partially due to improvements in strength, some of it is also attributed to neurological adaptations. The more familiar you become with the exercises, the stronger your mind/muscle connection becomes as new neural pathways are forged in your brain. Even if your strength gains plateau, you can still continue to refine your technique with persistent practice.

The specificity principle is part of the reason why newcomers to rings and parallettes will commonly struggle with basic exercises even if they're capable in other contexts. It's also a big part of why it is good to vary your training. If you only do one workout program forever, you will only get good at those specific exercises. In order to be well-rounded, it's important to keep your body from getting too comfortable with any particular routine.

ANALYSIS PARALYSIS

Admittedly, this is a lot to consider, but try not to get overwhelmed. Like most things in life, you probably aren't going to design the perfect program for yourself on your first attempt. That doesn't mean you shouldn't start.

Too many people get caught up in the theoretical end of programming and forget that without actually following through on those plans, they have no value. A poorly designed program that is well executed will yield superior results over a seemingly great plan that is not adhered to. Good things come to those who train.

There will inevitably be some trial and error in order to find what works best for you, but that's part of the learning process. Furthermore, individual factors like age, gender, previous exercise experience and lifestyle will make each situation unique. You need to stick to one plan for at least a few weeks to tell how well it is (or isn't) working.

So deal with what's actually taking place rather than any predetermined hypotheses you may have brought to the table. Pay attention and trust your powers of observation.

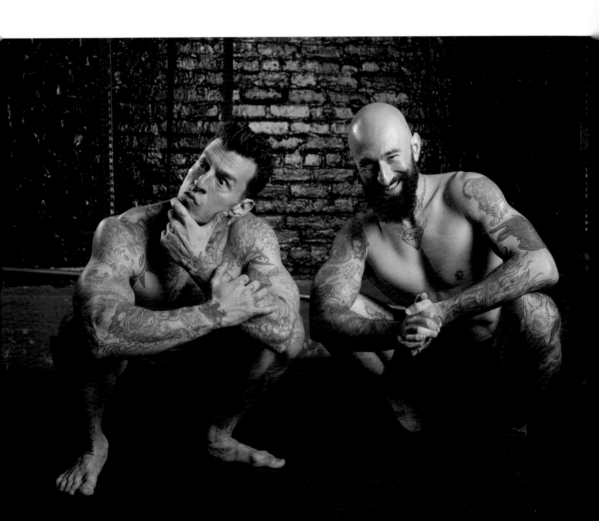

FLOW WITH IT

As you get more advanced, you can begin to explore stringing exercises together in a continuous flow. Parallettes and rings lend themselves very nicely to this style of training. By practicing the transitions between various exercises, you will build better control and learn to move your body in unique ways.

You already have some experience with the following basic parallette flows:

BASIC FLOWS

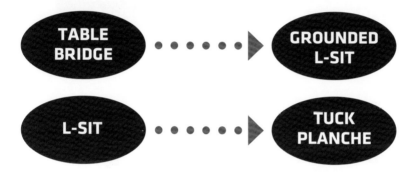

Here are some advanced flows you can experiment with after you have completed the program:

PARALLETTE FLOWS

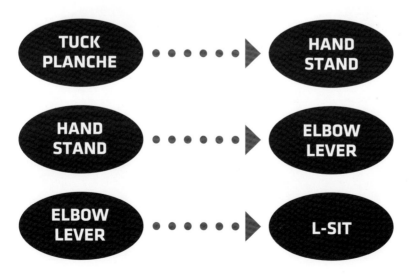

RING FLOWS

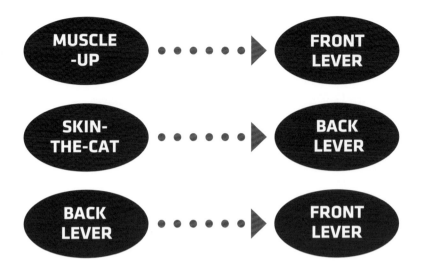

You can even combine longer flows together. For example:

EXTENDED PARALLETTE FLOW

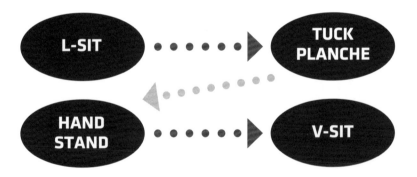

EXTENDED RING FLOW

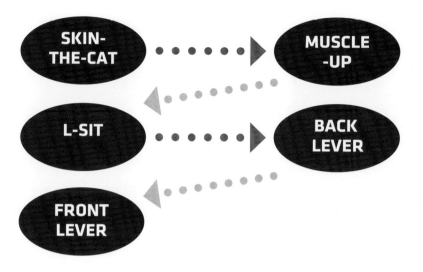

There are many other flows. Use your creativity and strength to come up with your own sequences.

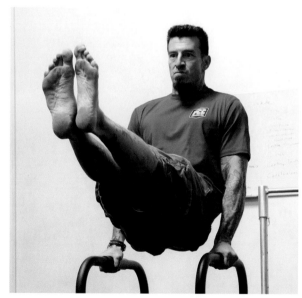

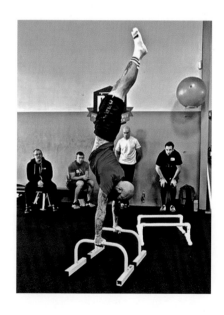

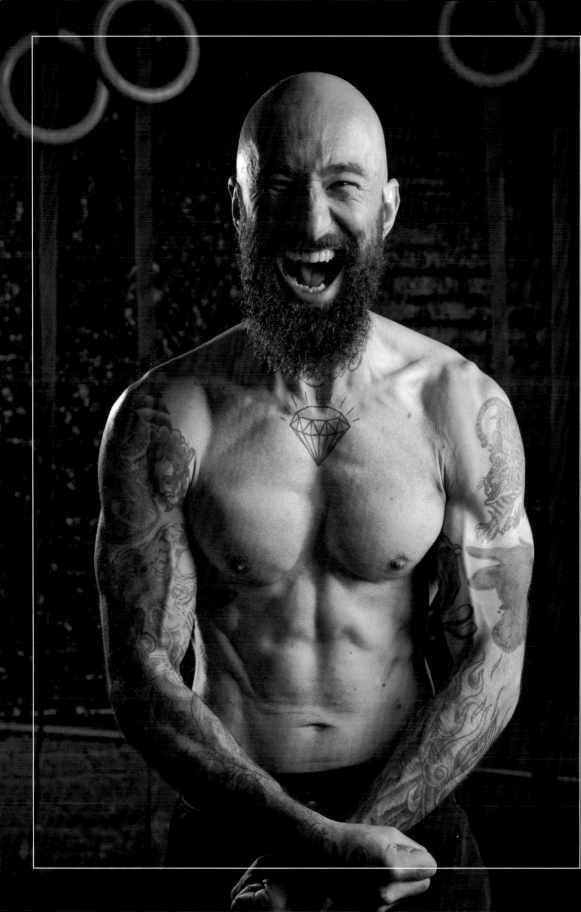

Ask AI

Can you really build muscle with just bodyweight training? Don't you need to lift weights if you want to get jacked?

Yes, you can really build muscle with just bodyweight training. You do not need to lift weights. Regardless of the resistance, the mechanism behind all forms of effective strength training remains the same: You break down your muscles by forcing them to work harder than they are used to, then you give them time to rebuild and recover. Your muscles don't care if the resistance is coming from your own bodyweight or an external load. All that your body knows is that you're tearing down your muscle fibers, so they need to rebuild, adapt and become more efficient at producing force.

Then why are some people who lift weights so much more muscular than you?

You know how everyone has eyes, a nose and a mouth, but we all still have unique faces? Well the same is true of our bodies. We all have the same muscles in the same places but everyone's muscles look a little different. For some reason, it's easy for people to accept that I have a big nose due to my genetics, but the same people often have a hard time wrapping their heads around the fact that my muscles are shaped the way they are due to genetics more than any other factor.

Just to be clear, this doesn't mean that anyone is genetically incapable of getting in great shape—we are all capable. It just means that some of us have a greater potential for mass than others. Everyone can gain muscle, but we don't all have the potential to look like Arnold.

In fact, most people who lift weights don't look like the guys on the cover of Flex magazine either. Look around any commercial gym. I guarantee you most of the people there are fat or skinny or both, and they're probably lifting weights.

Proportions can throw off our perceptions of size, too. Some of these guys aren't as big in person as they look in photos. If someone's waist is smaller than the sum of the circumferences of their arms, then they are going to look jacked even if they only have 14 inch biceps.

Also keep in mind that when someone is lean, they will look more muscular because their definition is not obstructed by adipose tissue. Lighting can also play a big role in how muscular someone appears.

And of course, let's not forget about steroids. Pro bodybuilders take steroids. That doesn't mean you can't get big without them—you can—if you eat right, train hard and have the genetics. But you probably can't get as huge and shredded as a pro bodybuilder without taking steroids.

So try not to compare yourself to anyone else. It's better to simply focus on being the best YOU that you can be. It's important to be ambitious, but please be accepting of yourself even if you aren't as huge as Arnie (or even ol' Al).

Are these workouts only for men or can women do this program as well?

Women can absolutely do this program! Though in general, men are biologically predisposed toward a greater propensity for upper body strength than women, strength training is very much a unisex pursuit. That said, women may find that they progress slower with some of the upper body movements, but we all have the potential to perform these exercises if we are dedicated to the training.

Should I do these workouts as a circuit or is it better to perform all sets and reps of one exercise before moving onto the next?

We wrote this program intending for the exercises to be performed in sequence as written. This means we want you to complete all sets and reps of a given exercise before moving ahead to the next one. We feel that this will yield the best results as far as gains in strength and technique are concerned.

However, some people may prefer to do these workouts as circuits. There are potential advantages to doing so, such as saving time, as well as placing more emphasis on endurance. Ultimately, it's up to you to decide which approach is better suited to your situation.

Do I have to do the exercises in the order that they are written? What if I want to work my legs first?

The workouts are written in the order that we find most beneficial, but you can change up the sequence however you think is best. Remember, it's okay to modify the program based on your own experience and preferences.

Can I split the workouts up and do half of it in the morning and half later in the day? Or what if I wanted to do the parallette workouts and the rings workouts on different days entirely?

Yes, you can do the parallette exercises and the rings exercises separately if that works better for your schedule. It's not ideal, but it's definitely better than skipping out on any of them entirely. Get those reps in whenever you can!

How do I know if I am performing the exercises correctly?

First things first, be sure to carefully read the exercise descriptions and look closely at the illustrative photos. From there, a good way to objectively assess yourself is to video your workouts and watch them back with a critical eye.

Taking a video of your training session isn't just for showing off on Instagram. You can learn a lot by watching yourself! In fact, you may find that what you think you are doing and what you are actually doing are two very different things. Watching a video of yourself can help you accurately assess your form and (hopefully) fix your mistakes. Reviewing your video can also give you something to do while you're resting between sets.

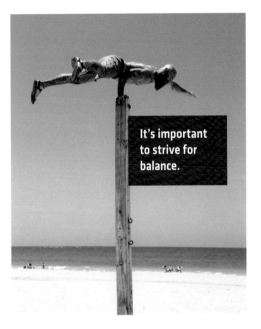

It's important to strive for balance.

I'm advancing faster with certain exercises than others. Is it okay to mix and match different parts of the different levels of the program?

Sure! You may progress faster with some things than others so it's fine to personalize the program. You may find that you are ready to move on to more advanced parallette exercises but are still working with beginner rings progressions; others may experience the opposite. Just be careful not to fall into the habit of only training your strengths while ignoring your weaknesses. It might be more fun to train the exercises that you are better at, but it's also important to strive for balance.

I just did my first training session and I can't believe how sore I am! Is everything okay?

Sometimes when people are new to this type of training, it can greatly shock the body. Don't worry—this is a good thing! However, following your first workout (or your first workout in a long time), it's not unheard of for muscular soreness to linger for an entire week or more, so don't be alarmed. If you need additional rest days, then take them. You may find that during the first week of each level, you may need more recovery time due to introducing new movements into your regimen. This is fine.

It hurts when I do a certain exercise. Should I keep doing it anyway?

No. Pain is a signal from your body that whatever you are doing is causing harm. However, some discomfort is to be expected during intense exercise. It's important to recognize the distinction.

If you are experiencing actual pain—it shouldn't be too hard to tell the difference—then you may be performing an exercise incorrectly, attempting something that is outside of your current capabilities and/or you have an injury or ailment that is causing the problem. Do your best to make adjustments accordingly. If you are unable to find a solution, seek the help of a medical professional.

Is it okay if I combine this program with other workouts?

We wrote this program to give those who follow it a thorough, full-body overhaul without the need for any additional exercise, but the program can be modified to include other exercises as well. For example, you could go jogging or cycling on your days off from Next Level Strength if you aren't really the "rest day" type. You could also do these workouts only once or twice a week instead of the recommend 3-4 times a week, while doing other workouts on your other strength training days.

You can even use this book as a supplement to an existing program or regimen. If you want to just pluck out a few exercises that you like, then feel free to try them in your workout however you see fit. I'm a big believer in personal experimentation and I encourage you to follow your own curiosities. You don't have to follow the program exactly as written if it's not ideal for your current situation. You have my blessing to make modifications based on your own firsthand experience.

I would, however, advise against doing this program as written while simultaneously following another strength program. Training is definitely important, but rest is important, too. Besides, you probably wouldn't be able to follow either properly if you were doing them both at the same time.

How should I breathe when performing these exercises?

In through the nose, out through the mouth. Moreover, it is commonly suggested that inhaling during the eccentric (lowering) phase of an exercise and exhaling through the concentric (lifting) phase of an exercise can help generate the most power. But some people prefer to do the opposite. There is no proven consensus on which method will work best for all people in all situations. I encourage you to try both ways and see what feels better for you.

What about breathing during isometric holds like L-sits?

Just try to breathe as normally as possible and make sure you do not hold your breath, although you may find yourself breathing harder than normal simply because you're exercising.

When I try to hold an L-sit, I get muscle cramps in my quadriceps. What's the problem, lack of strength or lack of flexibility?

What you are experiencing is very common. You're on the right track thinking that strength and flexibility are both potential culprits here. In fact, it's most likely a combination of the two.

In order to perform a proper L-sit, you need to have adequate range of motion in your hamstrings as well as ample strength in your quads and hip flexors. The tighter the muscles of your posterior chain become, the harder the muscles in front have to work in order to counteract them. I recommend practicing some old-school toe touches to help loosen them up before your next session.

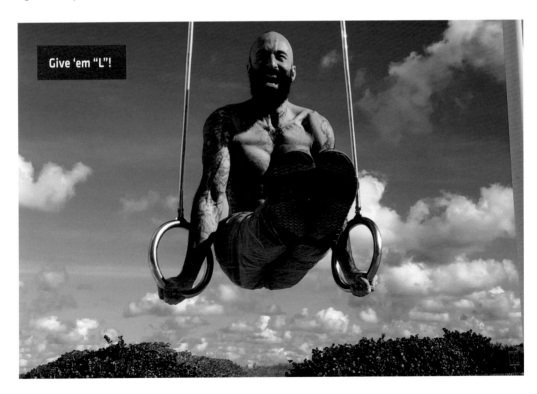

Give 'em "L"!

My ceiling is too low for me to set my rings high enough to fully extend my legs at the bottom of a pull-up. Is it okay if I bend my knees and keep them behind my back so that I can go all the way down?

Though it's not ideal, sometimes we're forced to work with limited space. If you find yourself needing to move your legs out of the way in order to fully extend your arms, I'd actually recommend reaching them in front of your body rather than behind. Reaching the legs forward will increase your abdominal engagement, while placing them behind the body will do the opposite. Try it both ways and see for yourself.

I read in one of your other books that I should grip a pull-up bar with my thumbs on the same side of the bar as my other fingers, but in this book you say to grip the rings with the thumbs wrapped around the opposite side. Why the difference?

Good observation! Due to the fact that rings are circular, most people find that it feels better to wrap their thumbs around the opposite side. I encourage you to experiment with different grips to find what works best for you.

The false grip hurts my hands and wrists. I've even got a bruise at the base of my palms. What am I doing wrong?

The false grip can be surprisingly challenging at first but you probably aren't doing anything wrong. When you train on rings, you work way more than just your muscles. You also strengthen your tendons, ligaments, bones, cartilage, and yes—even your skin! That bruising near your wrist is a sign that your skin is starting to toughen up. Try to see it as a badge of honor or a "battle scar" rather than a problem. With practice, the skin will become stronger and you will no longer experience that bruising.

Which is harder, a muscle-up on rings or a muscle-up on a pull-up bar?

Regardless of the apparatus, the most challenging part of a muscle-up is typically the transition from the pulling phase into the pushing phase. When you perform a muscle-up on a bar, this transition can be especially difficult, as you have to maneuver your body around the bar. When you do a muscle-up on rings, however, you can move your torso in between the rings, which most people find easier.

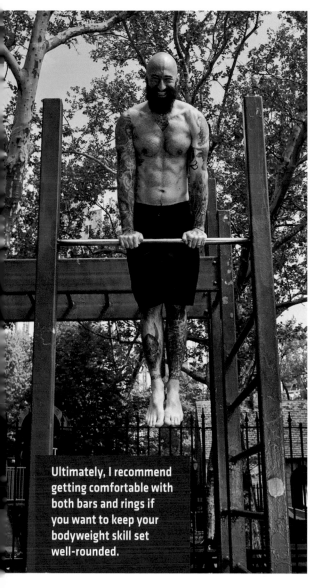

Ultimately, I recommend getting comfortable with both bars and rings if you want to keep your bodyweight skill set well-rounded.

While rings are less difficult to get around during the transition phase, they are unstable and therefore provide a unique challenge during the pulling and pushing phases. I've known people who learned the muscle-up on rings first, and then struggled to learn it on the bar, despite proficiency on rings. Conversely, I've known others who learned the move on the bar first, and then struggled to get it on rings.

So you see, it is not such a clear-cut case of one being harder than the other. There are some aspects of the bar muscle-up that make it more difficult than a muscle-up on rings and vice versa. Either way, the muscle-up is an advanced move that will take some trial and error to achieve. Ultimately, I recommend getting comfortable with both bars and rings if you want to keep your bodyweight skill set well-rounded.

How do I know when I have mastered an exercise and am ready to move ahead to harder progressions?

As a general rule, you should get comfortable with the basic versions from each family of exercises before moving on to more advanced progressions. That's why we suggest spending approximately 8 weeks on each level. This book is laid out in such a way as to guide you through the progressions, building to more difficult moves in the higher levels. We encourage you to take your time and embrace the journey.

To be clear, there is no such thing as true mastery. Having an ideal to strive for is helpful, but perfection is an illusion. Aim to do your best, but don't get frustrated if things continually need refinement.

Should I still work out if I am sick?

As a general rule, if you feel like you are starting to come down with something, I would not recommend training that day, even if you have a workout scheduled. The best way to keep sickness at bay is to rest, stay hydrated and avoid stress. Adding the burden of a training session to the mix will only further tax your immune system, making it more likely that you will succumb to illness.

If you are currently sick, I recommend resting until you feel better. My one caveat is that if you're starting to feel better and you're eager to get back to training, a light workout might be helpful. Just take it easy. Keep your intensity to 50% or less of what you would normally do. This will help get your blood flowing and encourage deep breathing, which can help your recovery.

Furthermore, the best way to deal with training around illness is to not get sick in the first place. Ample sleep, proper nutrition and stress management are all crucial for avoiding ailments. If you find yourself getting sick more than once or twice a year, chances are that you are not taking proper care of your body.

I've been following the program for a while but I feel like I'm not making progress anymore. I've been stuck on the same workout for almost a month! What can I do to bust through this plateau?

When you're new to training, it's amazing how quickly you can see improvement. But anyone who's trained consistently for long enough eventually sees their progress level off. It's simply a matter of diminishing returns.

Your second workout might feel a lot better than your first one, because two workouts is twice as much exercise as one. But your 100th workout might not feel much different from workout number 99, even though they are both only one more session than the previous one. Going from zero to one—nothing to something—that's the big chasm. Everything after that makes less and less of a difference.

Also remember that there are ways to gauge your development other than adding reps. If you've been training consistently, it is likely that your body awareness and exercise technique are improving. Pay attention to see if you feel more in control of your movements. Try not to get too hung up on the numbers.

Have you ever experienced tendinitis? What did you do to help fix it?

I have and it sucks! Sometimes the solution is simply to take a few days or a few weeks off from training. If you're still relatively young and/or your tendinitis is not very severe, this may be all that is required. Just be careful when you start back up to take a bit more rest in between intense workouts.

Heat can also be helpful. Hot tubs, saunas and heating pads all promote circulation, which promotes healing. Cold exposure can help, too. Whether in the form of cold showers, ice baths or ice packs, the healing powers of the cold are undeniable. (Check out "Winter Warrior" on page 160 for more information.)

The key to longevity is to strive for slow and steady progress over the long haul, while occasionally swapping between periods of higher intensity training and lower intensity training. So if you need to scale it back for a little while, we encourage you to do so.

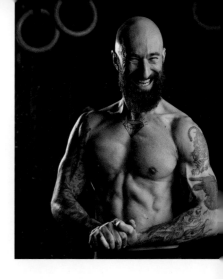

It seems like you are always smiling! How do you stay so positive?

Sometimes people are under the impression that I never think negative thoughts or feel lousy, but that's certainly not the case. I experience the same spectrum of emotions as anybody else. I'm no stranger to sadness, anger, guilt, jealousy and other negative emotions. In spite of that, I've managed to cultivate an overall positive mindset that's helped me both as a fitness coach, as well as in my own personal pursuits.

You see, thoughts arise on their own—we can't really control what we think—but we can make a decision whether or not to attach ourselves to a thought. In that sense, staying positive is a choice, and it's also something that you can get better at with practice.

When you find yourself thinking negative thoughts, sometimes it helps to try to take a step back and get objective about the situation. The human mind has an amazing ability to identify problems. But when there aren't any real problems, sometimes we find a problem where there isn't one. It helps to recognize that this mechanism exists within the brain so that we don't succumb to it too often.

I make it a point to remind myself on a regular basis how lucky I am to have basic necessities like food, running water and a roof over my head. Then I think about my family and friends and how lucky I am to have them. Even still, those negative thoughts can creep back. It's just part of being human. Sometimes you need to let yourself feel bad in order to move forward. Ignoring those feelings isn't always the answer. In fact, it can make things worse.

When we ignore a problem, it tends to grow until it gets to the point where it simply cannot be avoided. So we need to be honest with ourselves and confront those feelings head on, which can be very difficult. However, it is often the most difficult tasks that lead to the most satisfying outcomes. The harder we work toward accomplishing an objective, the better we feel when it's behind us.

Beyond that, finding things that you enjoy and immersing yourself in them can help give your life more meaning. Too often, people spend most of their waking life doing things they don't enjoy. It's no wonder so many people experience chronic depression. If you hate your job, find a better one. If you're in a toxic relationship—leave! You don't have to be unhappy.

And of course, let's not forget that exercising helps alleviate stress and anxiety, and so does having some sort of creative outlet. That's part of why I keep working out and writing!

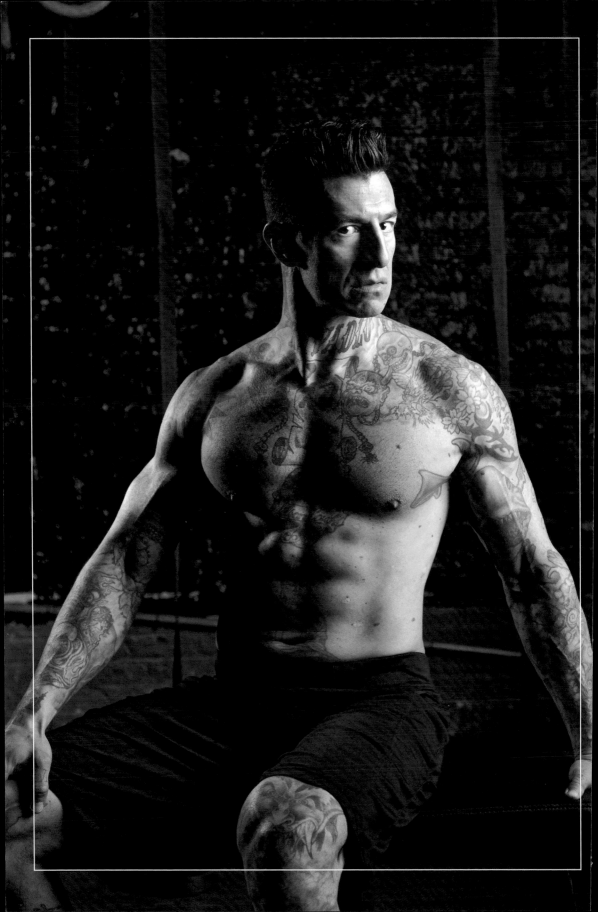

Danny's Dos and Don'ts

DO COMMIT

Back in Brooklyn in the 1990's, we used an expression to describe when someone was truly committed. We called it "D.F.L."

D.F.L. means "Down For Life."

Fast forward a few decades to May, 2017. At this time, a gentleman named Salim Attye flew all the way from the Republic of Senegal to London, England in order to attend a Progressive Calisthenics Certification (PCC) instructed by my brother Al Kavadlo and myself. This young man knew the immense value of attending the PCC course, which covers all the calisthenics basics like squats, push-ups, and pull-ups, as well as the more advanced "money" moves like floor holds, human flags and muscle-ups. In addition to the technical information about exercise, progression and programming, our curriculum is based in an experiential teaching methodology. In other words, we focus on real hands-on practice where every participant is involved in every step of the way. The feeling—physically, mentally and even emotionally—of attending this workshop is unparalleled. At all PCCs, personal records are set, lifelong friendships are made and wisdom is exchanged.

Leading up to PCC weekend, Salim understood the need to take his training seriously. After all, change does not happen hastily. It is a process that takes time, and the only way to be effective is to stay the course. During the workshop, it was clear to us that he'd practiced his moves. He'd invested energy, effort and, perhaps most importantly, hours.

As a personal trainer, I encounter people every day who claim they want to change their lives and bodies. The ones who actually mean it decide to commit. We all have twenty-four hours in a day, 365 days in a year and 1,001 excuses we can invent for skipping a workout,

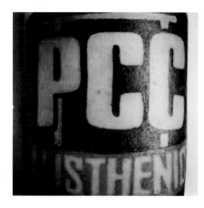

bailing on an event or straight up lying to ourselves. In life and fitness, there are things you do and things you do not do. If something is important, then you prioritize it and give it the resolution it deserves. If it isn't important, you don't. It's very obvious and simple. Without commitment, real, long-term results cannot be accessed. It's important to respect this. My friend Salim sure did.

Next time we saw him, he had the PCC logo tattooed on his skin. Now that's commitment! He is D.F.L.

DON'T AVOID HARD WORK

It's true that commitment is a key part of the equation, but still, we must acknowledge that words alone (even when accompanied by tattoos) will not take you far. Only execution will. So don't be afraid to work hard—and at times even suffer—in order to move forward.

When I was in my early thirties, after a series of unusual careers including touring musician, clown at kids' parties and spring break emcee, I opted for my strangest vocation yet: Personal Trainer. This was shortly after my son was born and I was dead-set on getting off the road and switching careers. Although I'd worked out for most of my life, aside from occasionally dragging some of my non-workout buddies to the gym with me and showing them the basics, I had absolutely no experience as a fitness professional.

Given my life circumstances at the time, including a new child and a new mortgage, I had a lot at stake. There was no choice but to take action!

I got hired at a big box gym and let my boss know that I'd take every single lead available for a prospective client anytime, anywhere. I volunteered to train anybody who was even *slightly* interested. I showed up earlier than anyone else and stayed later. Even though it wasn't in my job description, I re-racked weights, picked up people's used towels and even sold training for other trainers. I may not be the sharpest tool in the shed, but I'll outwork anybody. With this ethic, in time, I built my clientele.

Eventually I was promoted to Personal Training Manager at the largest club in the company. I was now responsible for a staff of forty professional trainers and an annual sales goal of 2.4 million dollars. More than ever, I had to go above and beyond the basic job requirements in order to be successful. Put away weights and towels? Fuhgeddaboudit! Now I took out the trash, watched infants so their mommies and daddies could work out with my staff and even handled memberships sales. I worked my ass off in every aspect of my job (as well as the jobs of others) in order to accomplish the larger objective. This was not easy, but most goals are not easy (and many easy things are not goal-worthy). The company sales and training records I set in 2008 during the "Great Recession" remain unbroken to this day. Hard work pays off.

The same principles I applied to work also apply to workouts. You must put forth effort frequently and consistently. You cannot fake it. Physical training lives in a place where all that exists is integrity and purity. There are so many variables in life of which we have little or no control, but not when it comes to your body. If you put in the hours and the effort, diligently and consistently, you WILL get results. Everyone will. This is indisputable. That's part of what makes it great.

No job in or out of the gym is too big or too small. When something needs to be done, you do it. That is how you get results. These seemingly small steps will help you realize the overall goal. Training is an active process and needs to be prioritized. You will have to adjust your schedule to make time for your workouts. This is 100% within your control and there are enough hours in the day to get it done. Clear your mind and attend to the task at hand. Those ups ain't gonna push themselves!

DO EAT GOOD FOOD

The food we choose to eat is the most important decision we can make regarding our health. That's right—even more so than exercise! We've all heard the cliché "You can't train your way out of a poor diet." Well, it's true. No amount of training can offset a steady stream of dietary disasters. Putting quality, whole ingredients in our bodies gives us better fuel for living a more vital and enjoyable life than snacking down shoddy substitutes.

Generally speaking, the only way to be sure of what you're eating is to prepare your own food. For this I recommend keeping things simple. Stick with fresh fruits and vegetables instead of those in a can or box. Buy fresh dairy and animal products from local sources whenever possible and avoid packaged food products. If you find the latter to be difficult, then at least read the labels on the packaging. If there are too many ingredients listed (or if the list reads like a science experiment) then stay away. Check out "recommended" serving sizes, too. Sometimes what we suspect is a single serving was intended to be several, leading us to eat more than we may think.

It's also good to avoid food products which make extensive health claims. I know that may sound counterintuitive, but the truth is that products boasting "low fat", "no sugar," or "gluten free" are usually no better (and very often worse) than the original counterparts. To render them appealing to the palette, questionable ingredients are often added to compensate for what's missing.

The best foods usually don't come in a printed package anyway.

There is a principle in food shopping known as "the perimeter rule," which means that the fresher products are located on the outside aisles, along the perimeters of the market. This is because these foods expire quicker, so the inventory must be tended to more frequently. The stuff in the middle will probably outlast us all. Real food goes bad before long. Fake food products don't. For the record, I also consider supplements like protein powders, fish oils, liquid aminos and BCAAs to be fake foods. I wouldn't trust a protein bar unless I made it myself!

In other words, less processed is generally better. Of course, this is the part when someone usually (and correctly) points out that almost everything we eat is processed to some degree. It's true. The beef I'm chewing on has been butchered and cooked. The wheat's been harvested, milled and threshed. I peeled this banana myself. So, yeah, I am not saying to eat only food that is *completely* untouched by man, simply to use a little common sense. There is a difference between the way a local farm-raised hen is processed and the way a chicken nugget assembled from a thousand mechanically separated animals is processed. By the same token, old-school sourdough bread containing only flour, water and salt is far superior to bleached-out, over-milled Wonder-style bread product. Think about where your food comes from. Adopting clean eating habits will provide you with superior nutrition and spectacular energy. I'll bet it will taste better, too.

Now that we're avoiding overly processed foods, there are still a few broad strokes we can apply in order to meet our optimal goals. These include consuming more vegetables (more vitamins, nutrients and fiber), drinking more water (increased metabolism and waste removal) and eating only when hungry. That's right; many times people kid themselves into thinking they're hungry when they are simply bored, eating out of habit or caving to a craving. If you're truly hungry then you'll gladly bite into a crisp, sweet apple. If that doesn't sound appealing, you may be munching for reasons other than hunger.

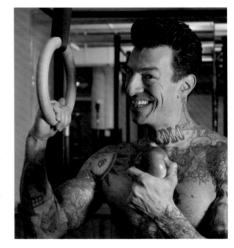

Most of us could also probably stand to consume less sugar (even organic cane sugar, agave nectar and other "natural" sweeteners, not just high fructose corn syrup). Be careful about drinking your sugar, too. Sodas, sweetened iced teas, and energy drinks, although sometimes billed as healthful (you know how I feel about health claims) are full of gratuitous sugars and other additives. Stay away.

Those are my biggest dietary recommendations. Nothing too complicated.

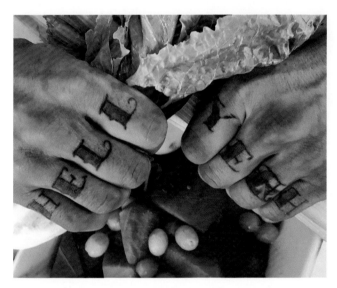

Personally, I eat much more balanced than most current "name" diets advise. Trendy memes like "Keto," "Vegan" or "Carnivore" place a gimmicky spin on eating by claiming that the secret to success lies in completely omitting entire food groups forever. Personally, I'm leery of any recommendation to omit all carbs, all animal products or all non-animal products, as those foods have been healthful staples of the human diet for thousands of years. By contrast, the obesity epidemic is only a few decades old.

Speaking of obesity, the only way to lose weight is to expend more energy (during exercise, daily activity and base metabolic rate) than you consume from food and beverages. This is sometimes referred to as a caloric deficit. A calorie is the unit we employ to measure the amount of heat energy we take in through food or "burn" from activity. Any time the latter is greater than the former over the long term, we get leaner. That's why so many eating styles and methods of weight loss (including the ones mentioned above) can work. By omitting entire food groups, they automatically restrict your total caloric intake, which will often lead to short term weight loss. However, there is a lot more to nutrition than simply reducing it to calories in and calories out. You need vitamins, minerals and other nutrients in order to be healthy. The nutrition plan listed ahead has proven successful for me and everyone I've ever met who has actually followed it.

That said, please note that I speak only from my own experience and I encourage you to experiment and find what works for you. I happily acknowledge that many people have gotten favorable results eating in other ways than I suggest and that is fine.

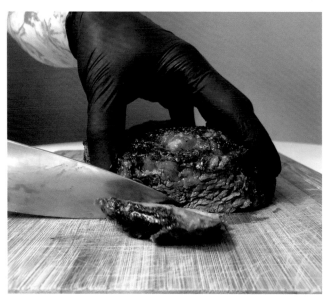

As a man in my forties who has experimented with just about every type of eating style, legal supplement and diet, I've come to the conclusion that keeping things simple instead of complicated has garnered the best results. And focusing on wholesome, minimally adulterated foods is better than counting calories. If you eat quality foods when you're hungry, you'll get full before you overeat. The fiber, enzymes and richness of such a diet is more filling than the starches, additives and sweeteners of diets that promote processed, "low calorie" offerings.

Usually when I discuss my personal way of eating, I simply say "mostly plants and animals." For you, my friends, I'll get a bit more specific. This is what I eat:

VEGETABLES & FRUITS:

Crisp greens (lettuce, kale, broccoli), hearty roots (carrots, beets and, YES, I eat potatoes) and vital stalks (celery, leeks) are all fair game here. So are apples, bananas, lemons, cabbage and peppers. I put fresh herbs like ginger, garlic, cilantro, parsley and lemongrass in this category, too, as well as beans and seeds. I usually eat vegetables and fruits at every meal, every day and they make up over 50% of my diet. I encourage as many colors, textures and flavors as possible. I also eat asparagus, Brussels sprouts and pears; to be clear, I am only listing a small sample of the almost endless amounts of foods in this and all subsequent categories.

MEAT, EGGS & DAIRY:

Fish, fowl, beef, lamb and all animals fall into this group, as well as eggs, milk, cheese, butter, cream and many others. The essence and vitality, as well as the complete proteins found in animals cannot be replicated. I also suggest eating organ meats, bone broth and marrow to get the densest nutrition and flavor. I eat meat almost every day.

NUTS & LEGUMES:

Foods like cashews, peanuts and almonds, just to name a few, are nutritionally dense and protein packed. They are excellent for snacking. Nut butters are great, too, but check the ingredients label for added sugars and emulsifiers. It shouldn't contain anything more than the nut itself and perhaps a dash of salt.

GRAIN PRODUCTS:

Bread, pasta and rice are the big three from this category, but there are others. They provide slow-burning fuel as well as ample nutrition. It is also very easy to overindulge on these calorically-dense foods. I recommend consuming them with caution as whatever is not burned off will be stored as fat. I generally keep consumption of grain products to about 3-4 times per week. I get my carbohydrates mostly from starchy vegetables like corn, squash and potatoes.

FATS & OILS:

I make it no secret that I enjoy olive oil, peanut oil, butter, grapeseed oil, hog fat, chicken skin and much more. Again, it comes down to quality. The fresher, the better. Fat is an essential nutrient and eating fat is not the same as being fat. I eat fat just about every day.

FERMENTED FOODS:

Sauerkraut, kimchee, miso, yogurt and pickles are all examples of the many fermented foods consumed around the world. Not only are these foods delicious, they have been shown to improve gut health and digestion. Just watch out for the added sugar in most commercial yogurt.

SUGAR:

Yes, I said we can all stand to eat less sugar, but nothing has to be avoided 100% of the time. Life is meant to be lived and loved. If we ever find ourselves in a state of deprivation or misery, then we need to adjust our attitude. Food should be a source of joy and never despair. It's okay to have a cookie or two, just not ten of them. And not every day. It's the "90/10 Rule" — If you're eating well 90% of the time (or even 80%), you can deviate for the other 10% (or 20%). Just be honest and real with yourself.

In other words, eat a balanced diet.

DON'T BE AFRAID TO GO WITHOUT

A balanced diet doesn't just mean that you eat a proverbial palette of diverse foods and food groups like I listed earlier. It also means managing the overall relationship you have with food. You see, many people (justly) have no problem occasionally partaking in some dietary decadence. However, unless you counter the days you go overboard with days of deliberate restraint, on a long enough timeline, the situation is likely to get out of control.

In other words, if you *ever* overeat, which we all do on occasion, there should also be times when you undereat. After all, it can't be Thanksgiving every day. In fact, it shouldn't be Thanksgiving *any day*, unless there are also days when you simply go without. That's the balance.

We live in a society where we almost never go without. If we want food now, we can use an app to order any cuisine we want, whatever time we choose. At the risk of being unpopular with the kids, I strongly feel that *NOT* getting what you want every single time you want it isn't such a bad thing. In fact, it's good. This is especially true with food—sometimes we need to go without. I'm talking about fasting.

The concept of fasting refers to voluntarily limiting or abstaining from food. It is a somewhat open-ended definition and can therefore be practiced in different ways. Fasting gives your digestive system (not to mention your liver and kidneys) a break, allowing you to "reset" your metabolism. You'd be surprised how much backed up waste we're carrying around in our guts all the time. By not cramming down food for a day or more, we can finally empty out. That's why the words "fast" and "cleanse," though not exactly the same, are often used interchangeably.

Other benefits of fasting include fat loss, improved metabolism and a boost to the immune system. Some experienced fasters claim improved internal organ function, though there is insufficient scientific data to conclusively say one way or another. Either way, the following is indisputable: When your body is truly fasted, you will feel incredible—energized, and centered, with a heightened level of focus.

To be clear, of course your body needs food. Protein, fats and fiber, along with vitamins and minerals are necessary and should be consumed on all normal, non-fasting days. But a fast is temporary. That's the point. It is a break from normal eating and is not intended to be sustained.

It's important also to note that part of Danny's Formula for Success is preparation. Just as you wouldn't try a muscle-up if you've never touched a set of rings or a pull-up bar in your life, you shouldn't jump into a fast if you've never before implemented dietary restrictions.

If that's the case, then instead of fasting, try just starting with a day or two where you eat only vegetables, fruits, nuts and seeds. This will help you assess if you are ready to fast or not. Also, try eliminating all beverages besides water, juice, herbal tea and black coffee. If this goes well, then you're ready to fast! Naturally, consult your doctor if you have any medical conditions.

There are several ways to approach fasting, and for success in any of them, you will have to come to terms with being hungry. Be prepared to exercise restraint. If it's your first fast, I do not recommend working out during this time, as your energy levels may be unpredictable.

Here are three popular ways you can fast:

WATER FAST

A water fast means that no food or beverages other than water are consumed for the duration of the fast. Even just one day requires great willpower. I do not suggest water fasting for longer than three days.

The beginning is usually the toughest and you may find that you are emotional or lightheaded. Stay the course. Throughout the fast, your mind and body will adapt and even accept. Believe it or not, after the first day or two, you will have more energy than you began with. You will become more awake and alert.

Sacrifice helps you become mentally strong. The human body is physically capable of going days, even weeks, without solid food, but most people never experience this because the notion of abstaining from food, even for one single day, is too terrifying to ponder. But this terror is birthed from the mind not the body.

At the conclusion of your fast (sometimes referred to as "breaking" your fast), ease back into your regular diet slowly. After not having eaten for a long time, it won't take much to fill you up. Also, you're likely to experience a new appreciation for the subtle complexity of every bite you eat. You'll be amazed at how incredible a single grape or green bean can taste. Your whole relationship with appetite and food will be altered, at least for a little while.

JUICE FAST

A juice fast is a more palatable way to get acquainted with fasting than a water fast because it does not completely eliminate all calories and flavors. You consume between 100-400 calories per day while juice fasting, compared to a water fast, where you'd consume none. Juice fasting also flushes your system with highly concentrated vitamins, minerals and enzymes which, although not filling, are incredibly satisfying.

When juice fasting, no solid solid food is consumed, and we drink only fresh vegetable and fruit juices, herbal tea, black coffee and vegetable broth. Have lots of water, too. Because we're avoiding sugar, I recommend juicing mostly vegetables (carrots, leafy greens & herbs are all great choices), rather than mostly fruits.

If it's your first time, try juice fasting for 24 hours. After a few tries, you may shoot for several days or even longer. I also suggest drinking many different juice variations. Getting your greens, reds, yellows, and purples not only provides a bouquet of rich and diverse flavors, it also delivers a boatload of nutrition.

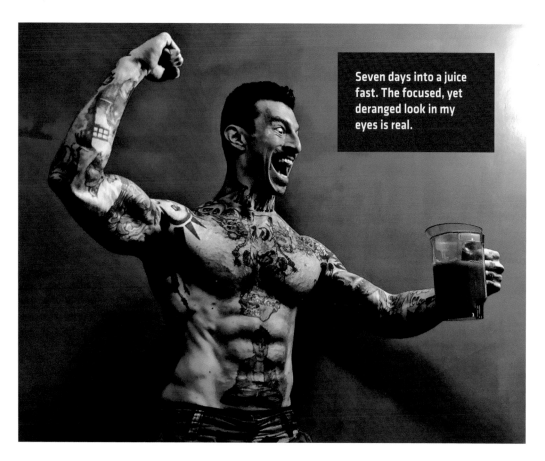

Seven days into a juice fast. The focused, yet deranged look in my eyes is real.

At the conclusion of a juice (or water) fast, your digestive tract will be empty and your organs less inflamed. It's likely you'll also be leaner, having burned off some superfluous body fat. But this short-term weight loss should not be a primary motivation. The fact that fasting resets one's appetite and cravings is far more relevant. This places us in a more advantageous position toward making mindful food choices in the future.

I.F.

The phrase Intermittent Fasting (I.F.) has gained a lot of press recently. Simply put, it refers to restricting how much food you eat, but basing the restriction on when you eat, rather than the foods themselves. This practice generally leads to a lean physique and desirable metabolic rate. Think about it: If you choose to eat, say, only from 1:00pm to 7:00pm for example, you're probably going to eat a lot less overall than you would without this time restriction. As we've discussed, eating less while maintaining the same activity level leads to weight loss.

Most of the time when people refer to I.F. they are talking about a daily food "window" of 8 hours or less (meaning a fast of 16 hours or more) as mentioned above. This really is not very long. Remember, it includes the time you're asleep. You can also do longer or shorter if you choose. In a sense, everybody does some sort of I.F. when they sleep at night and go hours without eating.

I.F. has other interpretations also and does not necessarily mean having a daily food window at all. It can also mean eating only one big meal a day, completely abstaining from food one or more days a week or spontaneously skipping meals. There are many ways to approach intermittent fasting and it doesn't have to be done the same every time, even for the same individual.

It's important to note that none of these fasts are rooted in longing or starvation. To me, quite the opposite is true. They nurture a greater appreciation, even respect, for food, flavor and all the sensory pleasures that go with it.

My personal eating practices could be described as intermittent fasting. I usually eat my first meal in the afternoon and seldom eat late at night. This is what I've done almost every day for the past 25 years, way before I ever heard the term "I.F." (I called it "skipping breakfast.")

I also do about 5-10 water fasts (one or two days each) per year, as well as 2-3 seven day juice fasts when I feel I've committed too many dietary transgressions. This keeps me lean and clean—and has intensified my love affair with food and cooking.

DO RECOVER

In fitness culture, we tend to emphasize the importance of diet and exercise, while often understating the large role that rest plays in our physical, emotional and mental wellness.

Those of us who have worked out seriously for long enough already know that without ample rest and recovery, one literally cannot grow. Sadly, sometimes well-meaning individuals are under the impression that muscular transformation happens during your workout, but in reality, it happens when you sleep. Nighttime is the right time for your muscles to repair themselves, not only from all your hard work in the gym, but also from day-to-day stressors like ultraviolet waves, pollution and other harmful toxins.

Getting adequate shut-eye allows your hormones to replenish themselves, improves overall cardiovascular health, decreases inflammation and helps your brain work properly.

Simply put, sleep improves brain function and alertness. You use rest and recovery to process the day's information and to create links, connections and memories in your mind.

Although the exact amount of sleep one needs varies from individual to individual (and even within the same individual at times), most people need seven hours or more per night.

To get a good night's rest, it is best to eliminate distractions. In other words, if the sunlight shines through your window at the crack of dawn, then hang blackout curtains. If your mind is racing, then put the phone away, along with all other electronic devices, an hour before bed. You'll be giving your eyes and brain some downtime. Perhaps more importantly, you'll be taking a break from the stimulating high that comes with every text, ping and ring. Get the TV out of the bedroom, too, for that matter, and never, ever eat or check email in bed. If that sounds outrageous, then that's all the more reason to give it a try.

Eliminating these distractions will help improve your quality of life across the board. As my longtime readers know, I am of the opinion that the bed is to be used for two things only: sleeping and making love.

DON'T BE IN A RUSH

When I was a kid, ordering a product through the mail took 6-12 weeks. There was no "30 minute guarantee" when you phoned in a food delivery either. And if we wanted music, we took a trip to the record store to buy it. Yes, records.

Now online purchases can be delivered the same day, you can order almost any food you want within half an hour (without even having to call!) and instant music downloads are delivered, well, instantly.

It's become a rare event in our modern world for anybody to experience a process *slowly*.

I'm not going for an Andy Rooney *60 Minutes* vibe here. I'll eagerly admit that these changes are by and large for the better. Most of our lives have been improved by the breakthroughs we've had these last few decades. From technology to communication to transportation, it's easier to be a human than it's been in any other time in history. But at the same time, it would be unrealistic to pretend that these miracles of the future come without a downside. Everything costs something and there are negatives to this revolution, too. One that comes to mind is that we sometimes feel like if it takes more than five seconds for an outcome to be achieved, then it's too damn long.

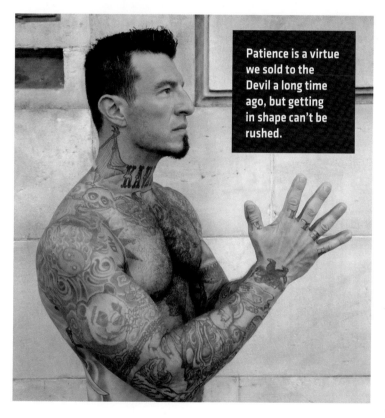

Patience is a virtue we sold to the Devil a long time ago, but getting in shape can't be rushed.

Patience is a virtue we sold to the Devil a long time ago, but getting in shape can't be rushed. That's part of the beauty of it.

Often in the realm of exercise, we expect physical advances to occur quickly, just like almost everything else this century. In reality, this is not entirely our fault. In fact, much of the fitness industry is based on perpetuating the lie of instant transformations. But please understand, if you've gotten out of shape over the past twenty years, it is somewhat unreasonable to think you can reverse it in just a couple of weeks. If you've never done an L-sit or a pull-up, then progressing to your first one will require consistent work for an extended amount of time. Don't expect an instant payoff.

Some things can't be rushed. The fact that physical changes cannot occur quickly is precisely what gives these changes so much value.

That's why Next Level Strength is arranged as a progressive program and not a quick fix. Because there are no quick fixes in training.

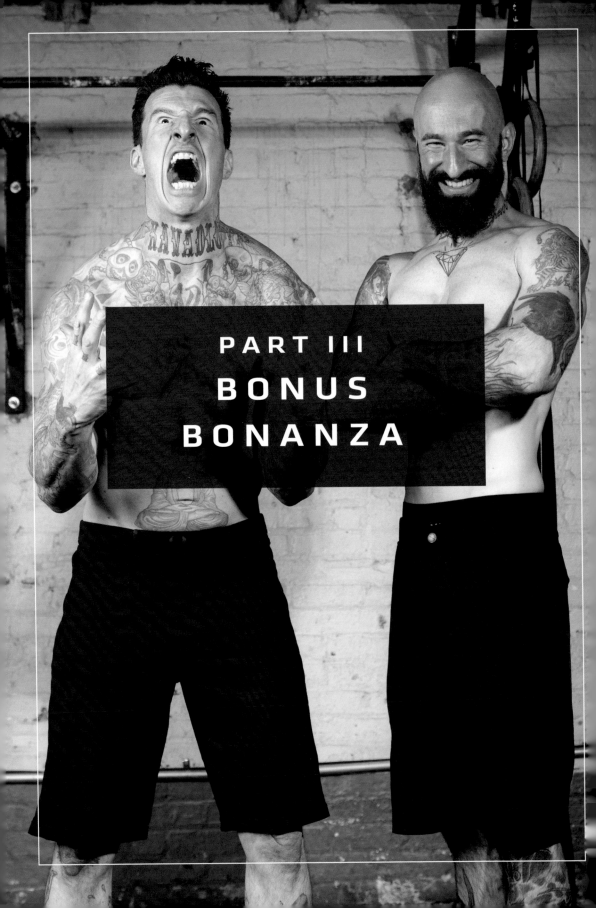

PART III
BONUS
BONANZA

Before and After

There's a saying that goes, "The only reason to look back is to see how far you've come."

While we appreciate the sentiment, it's one of those motivational sayings that sounds good at first glance but doesn't really hold up under scrutiny. There are other very fine reasons to look back. For example, reminding yourself of important lessons you've learned is a helpful way to avoid repeating the same mistakes again.

As writers, sometimes we reread one of our articles from years ago and find ourselves nodding along as though the words were written by someone else. With the amount of information we encounter on a daily basis, relying solely on memory is not the best method for keeping track of it all. Oftentimes, we must revisit important lessons repeatedly before they sink in on a deeper level.

What follows is a half dozen of our favorite articles from the last few years that have never before been seen in print. You may recall reading them, or they may be brand new to you. Either way, each of these articles pertains to a topic we get asked about frequently, and they're all filled with advice that's worth reading again and again.

In addition to sprucing up these articles for this book, we've also included brand new "Author's Insights" at the beginning of each one to provide a bit of additional commentary.

THE TOP 5 CALISTHENICS NEWBIE MISTAKES BY AL KAVADLO

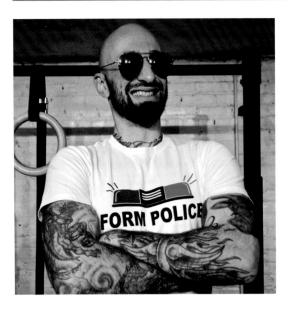

There's a guy at my local calisthenics park who likes to correct everybody's form. The other day I watched him criticize someone for failing to do the full range of motion during a set of dips. Though the critique was rude and inappropriate, he did have a point. The person in question was barely doing half of what I would consider to be the minimum range of motion.

Ironically, when the fellow who called him out went to do his own set of dips a few minutes later, he could barely perform half of the range of motion himself!

My reason for relaying this anecdote is not (just) to point out how obnoxious it is to offer unsolicited advice at the park or gym, but more to highlight how we're often terribly unaware of our own shortcomings. Pointing the finger is easy, but it takes character to turn the critical eye inward and be as objective as possible about your own training.

This applies to me, as well. Over a decade has passed since I began sharing workout videos on YouTube. But when I started filming my exercises, I was amazed to discover that a lot of the time what I thought I was doing, and what I was actually doing, were two very different things.

Though I've been training calisthenics for most of my life, I'm still continually learning. I've also coached thousands of others over the years and I've noticed a lot of the same issues tend to come up with beginners, and I sometimes see more experienced people making these mistakes as well.

Don't let the following pitfalls prevent you from making progress with your calisthenics training!

NEWBIE MISTAKE 1: NEGLECTING THE LOWER BODY

One of the most pervasive stereotypes about modern calisthenics practitioners is that we don't train our legs. Though I've been a longtime proponent of calisthenics leg workouts, this stereotype is not entirely unfounded. I've seen many folks focus so much on movements emphasizing their chest, arms, or abs that they forget about their legs entirely. This is true of many iron lifters as well.

Since your legs make up roughly 50 percent of your body, however, the fact of the matter is that if you don't have strong legs, you aren't really strong. The good news is that if you hit them hard, you only need to work your legs once or twice a week.

Start by mastering basic bodyweight squats—and doing lots of them. Then you can gradually progress your way up to single-leg pistol squats.

NEWBIE MISTAKE 2: FOCUSING ON MUSCLES OVER MOVEMENTS

In conventional strength training, it's common to try to isolate individual muscles or muscle groups with single-joint exercises like biceps curls or leg extensions, but with calisthenics our muscles work more effectively when we use them together. The sum is greater than the individual parts.

Don't get me wrong, there is more emphasis on certain muscles with certain exercises, but there is no such thing as true isolation in the world of calisthenics. Even an exercise like my beloved pull-up, which emphasizes the back and biceps, also significantly involves the chest and abdominal muscles. In fact, studies have shown that pull-ups actually recruit the rectus abdominis to a greater degree than traditional crunches and sit-ups.

The question "What muscle does this exercise work?" is so common in the strength-training world that many people forget the entire concept of muscle isolation didn't exist until bodybuilding rose to mainstream prominence.

When people ask me what muscles they work during a skin-the-cat or elbow lever, my answer is: "All of them!"

NEWBIE MISTAKE 3: RUSHING AHEAD

We all know how badass it looks to do a muscle-up or front lever, but you need to build the proper foundation before attempting any high-level calisthenics. Bodyweight training is among the safer strength training modalities, but any exercise is potentially dangerous if it is performed with poor technique or by a practitioner who is not properly prepared.

Establishing a solid baseline of strength is essential before moving ahead. Focus on getting comfortable with the basics before you experiment with anything more advanced. Your joints will thank you for it later.

NEWBIE MISTAKE 4: FAILING TO PERFORM A FULL RANGE OF MOTION

Though some lifters will intentionally perform partial reps, most folks who fail to complete a full range of motion believe they are going all the way up and all the way down. Like my form-policing friend at the park, oftentimes we feel like we are moving a greater distance than we actually are.

This is part of why it can be helpful to have a qualified trainer correct your form. If you can't find or afford one, recording video of your workouts is your next best option. Taking footage of your training can be a fantastic tool to help you assess your technique. You might see the full range of motion taking place in your mind's eye, but the camera can provide a more objective viewpoint.

NEWBIE MISTAKE 5: VALUING QUANTITY OVER QUALITY

While it's great to have ambitious training goals, focusing too much on reaching a certain number of reps in a given set—or even just a single rep that you're not quite ready for yet—can lead to sacrificing control and alignment. It's also another reason folks sometimes shortchange their range of motion.

Ironically, when you focus too heavily on the goal, you lose sight of what's actually happening in the moment. The truth is, you are much better off doing 5-6 strict, full range of motion pull-ups than 20 swinging half-reps.

You can still aim to get those 20 pull-ups, but if you are sacrificing form to get there, you're better off breaking them up into multiple sets in order to ensure that your technique remains intact. Take your time and focus on doing each aspect of every exercise with care and attention.

TRAINING, INC. BY DANNY KAVADLO

AUTHOR'S INSIGHT:

This article was originally published in 2014 on Bodybuilding.com under the title "Iron and Ink." Since I don't lift much iron in my own training, I made the executive decision to reinstate the original title here, along with a few other changes. Hellyeah, brother!

Tattoos and strength training go hand in hand. They conjure images of the tribal warrior, the sideshow strongman and the badass biker. They are both demanding at times, even brutal. But each one of these physical manifestations ultimately serves as a means to the same goal: making your body the way you want it to be!

This transformation transcends just the mere visual. When you're working out and sportin' ink, there's more to you than meets the eye. A powerful, sculpted body reveals many attributes other than just health, strength or attractiveness. The hidden meaning behind the fine physique is focus, sacrifice and dedication. Similarly, beyond the aesthetic of the tattooed body hides those very same qualities (as well as other meanings much of the time). Whether you're getting tattooed or getting diesel, you wear your results like a badge of pride. In both cases, you have to earn it

Oh yeah, there's one more big similarity: There's a lot of questionable information floating around about both. As someone with extensive ties in each community, it's not surprising that I'm often asked tattoo-related workout questions. Here are some of the ones I get the most:

Q: I want a tattoo on my arm, but I'm about to get HUGE! Won't the tattoo get stretched out?

A: The short answer is "No." You see, there are only certain areas from which your skin will stretch. The biceps/triceps area is not one of them. When your arms grow, it's the skin around the armpit that shows the evidence. For proof, take a look at the location of stretch marks on people who have had rapid changes in their weight. They're almost always around the pits. (And unless you're me, it's unlikely you will get tattooed there!) Even with substantial muscular growth, there is only so much your tattoo can realistically enlarge. A difference of a few inches in circumference would be astronomical on your arm's appearance yet would be virtually unnoticeable to the actual look of the tattoo. Whether you work out or not, skin changes over the years. That's just life. So if you want that biceps piece, just get it!

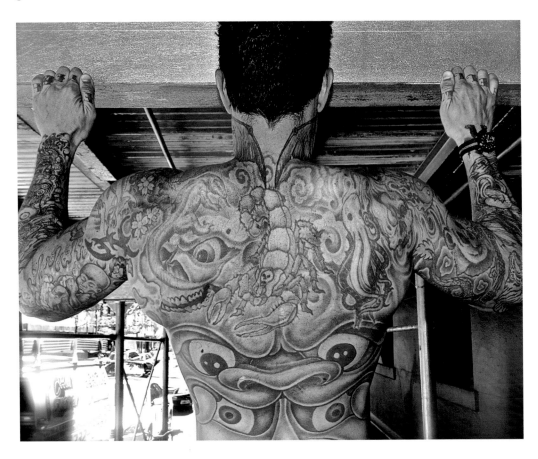

Q: "I heard tattoos need to heal. Do I have to stop training if I get one?"

A: Not necessarily. Think back to your last intense, heavy leg workout. Remember how you felt the next day? Did your legs need to recover? Well, just as your muscles require recovery after trauma, so does your skin. And while a tattoo is hardly a debilitating endeavor, it is still potentially taxing. Think about it. Your skin is getting stabbed by a needle and injected with ink thousands of times. It must heal. In fact, the way you take care of a new tattoo during the first 10-15 days is more important than the way you take care of it for the rest of your life. Just as your physique is not guaranteed when you leave the gym, that new piece is not guaranteed when you leave the studio. Keep it clean and moisturized and stay out of the sun.

I also recommend *not training* the freshly inked area for at least 2-3 days. This does not mean you need to stop working out altogether, just be smart about it. If you're healing a sleeve on your arm, then train your legs. If you just tattooed your thigh, then do some pull-ups. That said, regardless of any new tattoos, if you feel particularly debilitated, drained or tired, then listen to what your body is telling you. You are a better judge of your own recovery time than anything you read, including what you're reading right now.

Q: "I've been making great gains in the gym. If I get a tattoo, will it obscure my physique?"

A: Clearly, none of us who train hard want our tattoo work to outshine our work in the gym. Thankfully, the two make a perfect pair! One need look no farther than real life examples like Dwayne "The Rock" Johnson, Dave Bautista or Ruby Rose to see that bold, strong tattoos fit a bold, strong body like a proverbial glove.

When your tattoos conform to your own musculature in terms of shape, flow and size (I don't recommend getting a tiny piece on a big body part), it will enhance your hard work, not hinder it.

So invest the blood, sweat and tears to make your body the way you want it to be. Keep America beautiful. Work out and get tattooed! Hellyeah!

WINTER WARRIOR BY AL KAVADLO

Some of my earliest childhood memories are of playing in the snow. My mother would insist that I wear a coat, gloves and a hat, but I'm pretty sure I was ready to just dive in naked. After some resistance, I'd eventually bundle up as per Mom's orders, run into the yard, and roll around in the snow. Never once did I think about the temperature. I was having too much fun!

As an adult, I've continued to enjoy spending time outdoors doing physical activities, regardless of the weather. In fact, I've built my career around my passion for practicing calisthenics anytime, anywhere. I've also maintained my love for playing in fresh snow.

It's only recently, however, that I've begun to see how cold tolerance can be progressively trained the same way as your pecs or biceps. And there are just as many reasons to do so!

Here are a few to consider:

1 – INCREASED ENERGY

Though I'm not typically lacking in vitality, I do feel especially energized right after a cold shower. When the water hits my skin, it really wakes me up and gives my nervous system a jolt.

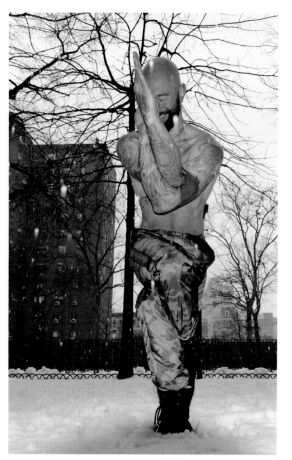

Science also shows that when the body is exposed to cold, it causes the capillaries to contract and blood is rushed away from the extremities in order to keep the internal organs warm. In the moments following cold exposure, the capillaries expand and fresh blood is returned to those areas. That's probably why I've had some really good workouts right after a cold shower.

2 – IMPROVED RECOVERY

When you're fired up, a cold shower is a great way to cool down. Though it may seem like a contradiction to my last point, cold showers are perfect after a workout, especially if you've built up a lot of body heat.

Cold exposure following an intense training session also seems to help relieve muscular soreness, which makes sense given the anti-inflammatory power of the cold. There's a reason it's common practice to put ice on a fresh wound or injury. The healing power of the cold is undeniable.

3 – THE ULTIMATE MEDITATION

The cold has an amazing way of bringing you into the present moment. It's pretty much impossible to daydream or think about anything other than the physical sensations you are experiencing while you are in the midst of cold exposure. All you can do is stand there, breathe and accept it.

So why aren't more people out there in the snow? For the same reason they don't exercise: We live in a culture that encourages comfort above all else. Just as children are often discouraged from physical activity—don't climb on those monkey bars, or you might get hurt!—we are also steered away from experiencing the elements. Over time, our willingness to change shrinks, and it becomes more daunting to start.

The biggest hurdle is, and has always been, your mindset. I'm sure you have a friend or two who thinks that you're crazy for working out at all. Keep that in mind if you start to think I'm crazy for spending time bare-chested in the cold.

Of course, you shouldn't jump into a shirtless workout in the freezing snow if you haven't been outside without a coat in 20 years. Just as it would be ill-advised to attempt a back lever on your first day of strength training, you should gradually ease your body into experiencing the cold.

I'm still a relative beginner at this, but I've already made progress in a short amount of time by using the following three techniques:

COLD SHOWERS

This is the perfect way to ease your body into experiencing the cold, because your shower is a controlled environment.

Start by taking a normal shower at a comfortable temperature and then at the very end, turn the faucet to cold and stay under the water for as long as you can. It will probably be a shock to your system at first, and you may begin hyperventilating. This is normal. Focus on slowing your breath and see if you can stay under the water for a full minute.

If you don't make it on the first try, that's fine. The first time I tried it, I barely lasted 30 seconds and found the whole thing to be quite unpleasant.

When it was over, however, I felt a powerful surge of energy which encouraged me to do it again the next day. After doing this daily for a few weeks, I'd conditioned myself to withstand several minutes under the cold water.

After a month or so of consistent training, you should be able to handle 5 minutes or longer without much trouble.

OUTDOOR COLD EXPOSURE

If your local climate is able to bring the cold, then this is an ideal next choice. All you need to do is steel your mind, go outside, and strip down to your shorts. If there is snow around, I encourage you to rub it on your chest and arms.

During your outdoor exposure, you can certainly move around in order to maintain your body heat. Yoga postures and calisthenics exercises like squats and push-ups are perfect, as they require no equipment and can quickly increase your internal body heat.

ICE BATHS

The final frontier of cold exposure is the ice bath. I wouldn't recommend trying this one until you are comfortable with the previous two. As the name implies, all you need to do is fill your tub with cold water, add ice and immerse yourself up to your neck.

If you are really hardcore, you can even seek out ice-cold water or cut a hole in a frozen lake and do your ice bath in nature, as Wim Hof has become famous for.

COLD WAR

Even after following Wim's teachings for the last several months and experiencing the benefits firsthand, it's still sometimes a struggle for me to turn the shower knob to the cold side. Occasionally there are days when I'm eager to feel the cold against my skin, but much of the time there's a voice inside my head trying to talk me out of turning that dial. And that's a big part of why I keep doing it.

Forcing myself to override the part of my brain that desires comfort has made me mentally stronger. Just like my calisthenics training, my experience with cold training has helped reinforce for me how to best approach potentially daunting tasks without getting overwhelmed. The key is to focus on breaking the bigger task down into smaller chunks.

On the days when I really don't want to feel the cold, I tell myself I'm just going to do 30 seconds. Once I get to that point, it's usually not hard to convince myself to endure another 30 seconds. After a minute, I try to convince myself to stay in for another minute. Sometimes it even starts to feel good!

There are days when I time myself and make sure I do a full 5 minutes. Other days I don't bother with the timer and just stay in for as long as I can handle. Of course, I do take a day off once or twice a week when I am feeling particularly dispassionate about experiencing the cold. Just like strength training, it's good to give your body a break from all that stimulation occasionally. Typically when I skip a day, I'm more eager to go for it the next time.

Also, keep in mind that hypothermia is real, and you definitely don't want it. Err on the side of safety when experimenting with cold exposure, and be on the lookout for symptoms of hypothermia, including intense shivering, lack of coordination, trouble speaking, confusion, or any loss of consciousness.

Just as patience and consistency with your strength training can make loads that you once considered heavy feel light, gradually building your cold tolerance a little each day can eventually lead to finding bliss in the frozen cold.

TRAINING AND DRINKING:
5 RULES FOR NOT COMPLETELY
RUINING YOUR GAINS BY DANNY KAVADLO

AUTHOR'S INSIGHT:

Most people I know who work out also drink alcohol (though not at the same time). When I wrote this article, originally published in 2018, it was important to me to discuss this subject in a realistic fashion.

At this time, I'd grown tired of the many gross oversimplifications I had read over the years. I was also getting sick of misleading talk from fitness professionals who have a "do what I say not what I do" attitude toward this subject. If there's one thing that gets under my skin, it's a hypocrite. People are complex and I have nothing to hide.

The opening scenario below really happened. It's what compelled me to write this.

Last Friday, I was crossing 5th Avenue, heading Eastbound on 23rd Street in the Flatiron District of Manhattan. I was en route to a personal training appointment, when a stranger approached me.

"Danny!" he exclaimed, "It's great to see you. You and your brother Al are a huge inspiration to me. I've been doing calisthenics for five years and I'm in the best shape of my life thanks to you!"

Wow! Stuff like this always makes my day. How could it not? I'll stop and chat with everybody and anybody when it comes to push-ups, pull-ups and pistols. Anything workout related, really. I'm happy to hear their stories and I consider myself lucky to have these opportunities.

After talking shop for a few minutes, the man surprised me with a rare demonstration of transparency. "Danny, I drink," he said solemnly.

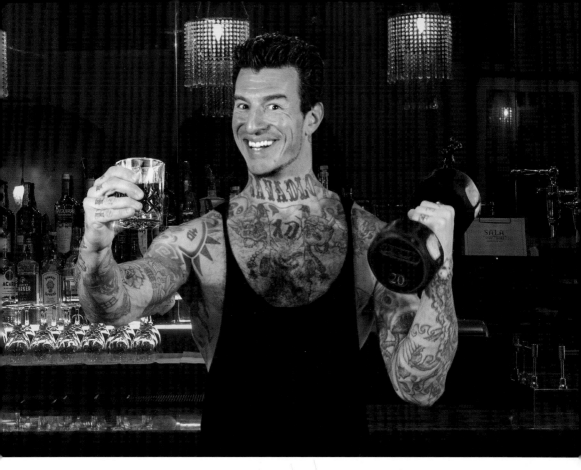

Perhaps the fact that we were perfect strangers enabled him to open up. Or maybe he knew that I'm the only guy in the game who dedicated a *whole chapter* to drinking in a book supposedly about abs. There are many possibilities. Who knows? He then followed up with the real question: "It's bad for gains, right?"

Hmmm, good question. I mean, it *is* bad for gains... Right?

WE LIKE SOME THINGS THAT ARE BAD FOR US

I know it's controversial to voice any perspective other than a loud, Nancy Reagan-style "Just Say No" when it comes to mixing booze and brawn, but that's not what you'll find here. Like many issues, this subject is more complicated than it may appear and cannot be dismissed with a simple, "It's bad. Don't do it." The fact is that an enormous number of people all over the world—*even healthy people who train hard, look amazing and feel fantastic*—like to drink.

It's true. Just about every culture on the planet—from the obscure to the ubiquitous—has discovered (and embraced) the process of making alcohol. Alcoholic beverages are incorporated into countless social, ceremonial and religious rituals, in almost every single civilization of modern mankind. Weddings or funerals, New Year's Eve or Passover, North America or South Africa, it seems that folks can't get enough of the hooch!

In fact, in the United States alone, the beer, wine and spirits industry grosses over 200 billion dollars annually, and that figure grows every year.

AN INCONVENIENT TRUTH

To be perfectly candid, it's a business I know well. The pull-up bar is not the only bar with which I have great experience. Prior to becoming a personal trainer in 2006, one of my many previous—and strange—careers was as a promotional marketer for a well-known liquor brand. (Think "Danny as Duffman"... not too far of a stretch.)

Long story short, I'd go on the road for months on end, traveling from "party town" to "party town," promoting the hard stuff. Believe it or not, despite my erratic, late-night schedule and sometimes self-destructive lifestyle, I still worked out four days a week and continued to get in better shape. Call it an inconvenient truth.

Obviously I'm well acquainted with the unfavorable effects that drinking can have on your fitness, and although I've scaled it back these days, I'm still a true believer that occasional use of alcohol *does not have to be a complete deal-breaker*. At least it hasn't for me. Sometimes seemingly contradictory notions can and do co-exist, and this is one of them. That said, it's important to go into it with your eyes wide open and not kid yourself about the downsides. Let's take a look at some of the known negatives:

DOWNSIDE 1: IT DEHYDRATES YOU

One of the main reasons for your throbbing skull and dry mouth the day after a big night on the town is because of dehydration. You lose much more water than you gain when you drink. (Ever notice how often you run to the bathroom?) Because there's not enough to go around, water that should go to the brain is redirected to other organs, hence that headache.

DOWNSIDE 2: IT CAN LEAD TO WEIGHT GAIN

Alcohol is not a carbohydrate, fat or protein. It's just alcohol. At seven calories per gram, it is probably the emptiest of calories there is. An average alcoholic beverage is anywhere from 100–200 calories or more. All these gratuitous calories, when not metabolized, will be stored as fat. Not the look you were going for when you started training, huh?

DOWNSIDE 3: IT CAN DISRUPT MUSCLE GROWTH

Not only does alcohol have zero nutritional value, some studies say it may even disrupt muscle growth. (Google it if you have a day or two to kill.) Of course, many studies are questionable, reporting only on "chronic" drinkers or even non-human subjects. That said, anyone who's taken 9th grade biology knows that alcohol is metabolized before other nutrients, blocking them from being absorbed. This can hinder protein synthesis.

DOWNSIDE 4: IT INTERRUPTS YOUR SLEEP

You need sleep so your body can grow, repair and get strong. One of the ways that alcohol can affect your gains is by interrupting your sleep, thus depriving you of much needed rest. Though some people claim to sleep better after a few drinks, the sleep that comes afterward is very poor in quality. Muscle is built when you recover. You do not want to stand in the way of that.

MIXED MESSAGES?

I'm in my mid-forties and I am far stronger, perform much better and have way more muscle than I did in my early twenties and I do occasionally drink. Why? Because I enjoy it and I'm confident I can do it right. I won't let it ruin my life—or my gains!

Clearly, there are certain adjustments you can implement to turn something that's bad for you into something that's *slightly* less bad for you. Follow these guidelines and you'll be helping yourself more than you can imagine, should you choose to both train and drink. It goes without saying that you should never workout while under the influence.

You already know my Strength Rules. Here are my Booze Rules:

RULE #1: CONSUME LOTS OF WATER

It is extremely important to drink plenty of H2O before, during and after cocktails. In addition to several glasses throughout the day for general hydration, I suggest also having one glass for every alcoholic beverage you consume. At night, sleep with a bottle of water close by so you have easy access. If your urine is dark, you need more water.

RULE #2: DRINK THE GOOD STUFF

I never understood how anyone would work their ass of in the gym, spend their hard earned money on quality food and then binge out once a week on low-end "well" liquor or cheap beer. Go for the good stuff! Like master chefs, craftsmen of finer wines and spirits pay careful attention to their ingredients—and even the soil from which they came—not to mention the proper production process. The essence of everything we put in our bodies matters, even when it comes to libations.

RULE #3: NOT ALL POTENT POTABLES ARE CREATED EQUALLY

This may rub some people the wrong way, but my personal policy is "No mixed drinks, no beer, no exceptions." Most mixed drinks are loaded with sugar, sweeteners and chemicals. If you need a mixer, use club soda. Popular "hard" lemonades and ciders are some of the worst alcoholic beverages you can drink, as they combine the lowest quality alcohol with the lowest quality sugar. These beverages will put you on the road to weight gain faster than a glass of bourbon, or even vino. Beer is also packed with calories and your body absorbs it like a big can of sugar. If you choose to have a beer, do it for the flavor and stop after two rather than ten, as too many beers will turn your six-pack into a keg. Remember, anything your body does not use for fuel will be stored as fat.

RULE #4: DO NOT SUBSTITUTE ALCOHOL FOR SLEEP

Don't laugh. We've all seen somebody do this and we know what it looks like. Perhaps a coworker or classmate? Or maybe we've even done it ourselves? All I'm saying is, if you're going to tear it up, don't do it when you have to be at work at 7:00 am the next day. You need a full night's rest, probably even more to compensate. Enjoy your drinks, but not in place of sleep.

RULE #5: DON'T DO IT EVERY DAY

This is the most important rule on the list. Just like I say regarding dietary decadence, if you have a rule and you choose to cheat on a regular basis, then it is no longer cheating: it's your lifestyle. We are a product of our day-to-day habits. We have birthday cake at parties, and it's only okay because it's not the norm; it's the exception. I am generally fond of a good wine or whiskey, but like birthday cake (which I'm also fond of), if I consumed it every day, my life would become unmanageable.

CLOSING TIME

Adults make their own decisions. I am not here to tell you what you should or shouldn't do. I simply want to promote what I've observed to be true regarding training and drinking, as objectively as possible. In the world of wellness, fear-mongering tactics and absolutism often trump life experience, observation and common sense. Not for me, though.

Obviously, too much alcohol is toxic and can ruin your life, but there is no reason why a grown-up can't enjoy the ol' firewater from time to time and *still* be in great shape. If you are eating right 90% of the time, training hard and following my rules, then you've probably earned it.

As for the stranger who stopped me on 23rd Street, that's what I told him, albeit a shorter version. Cheers!

HOW TO TRAIN FOR A
ONE-ARM PULL-UP BY AL KAVADLO

AUTHOR'S INSIGHT:

The one-arm pull-up was one of the first advanced calisthenics exercises that captured my attention. It started as a curiosity, then eventually became an obsession. Even though I could do 20 strict pull-ups before I ever even thought to start training for the single arm version, it still took years of dedicated practice before I could perform a legit rep on both sides.

The one-arm pull-up is mercurial. You may feel like you're getting close some days only to find yourself seemingly back at the start the next time you practice. Even if you're already strong, learning the one-arm pull-up requires lots of patience and skill-specific practice. But if you want it badly enough, it is possible.

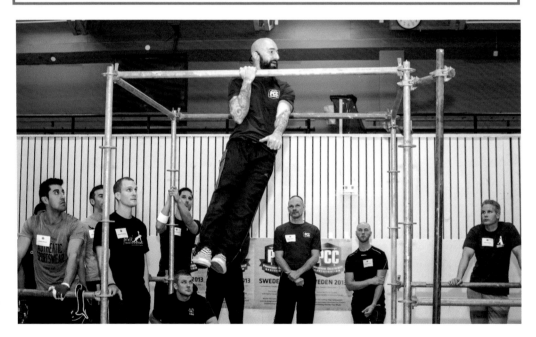

My one-arm pull-up journey began nearly a decade ago, immediately after I first saw one performed in person. Prior to that, I'd heard stories—legends, really—about the move, but never believed it was truly possible. The only time I'd ever witnessed someone do a pull-up with one hand was when the other one was wrapped around their wrist. Contrary to my initial expectation, however, a true one-arm pull-up is in fact possible.

In addition to achieving the one-arm pull-up on a few occasions myself, I've had the privilege of coaching some very strong people to perform their first one-armer as well. Though there are always many paths to any destination, I've concluded through my own trials and errors that the following techniques and tactics are the most essential, should you hope to one day tame this wicked beast of an exercise.

Before you begin working toward a one-arm pull-up, I urge you to spend plenty of time getting comfortable with the two-arm variety. Focus on getting to the point where you can perform at least 15 clean overhand pull-ups in one set without using momentum. Ideally, you should do closer to 20. This is the foundation for your one-arm pull-up.

HANG TIME

Once you've got that foundation, your next task is to get comfortable hanging with just one arm. This requires a serious amount of grip strength as well as strong, stable shoulders. If you can do 15 or more good pull-ups, you should pretty much be there already, but some dedicated practice is still necessary.

Focus on keeping your lats and shoulders engaged while you hang. In the beginning, just holding on for a few seconds may be very challenging. Eventually, you can work up toward longer one-arm hangs. A 30-second one-arm hang is a good target to aim for before moving ahead to anything more ambitious. If you have access to monkey bars or traveling rings, you can also practice swinging across them for additional single-arm work.

FLEX HANGS AND NEGATIVES

Just like a beginner can learn to do a two arm pull-up by performing a flexed arm hang at the top, the next step towards doing a one-arm pull-up is practicing a one-arm flex hang.

Start at the top position of a pull-up with your chin above your hands, then brace your entire body and carefully remove one arm. I suggest practicing this move with an underhand grip, as doing so allows you to keep your hand near the center of your body, which will make for better leverage. Though the burden of supporting your entire body weight appears to rest solely on one arm, your chest, lats, and abdominals are also an important part of the equation.

The first time most people try a one-arm flex hang, they immediately fall as soon as they take the other hand away. Don't be discouraged if that happens to you during your first few attempts. To help stay up, don't just think about your arm; focus on squeezing your whole body tight, especially your abs. You may find it helpful to keep your legs tucked close to your trunk when starting out. Eventually, work toward holding the position with your legs extended.

Once you can hold the top position of a one-arm flex hang for several seconds, you can begin to work toward a controlled one-arm negative. The idea is to start from a one-arm flexed hang, then carefully lower yourself into a dead hang with as little momentum as possible. Performing the eccentric phase of the one-arm pull-up is a great way to prepare your tendons and ligaments for the stress of the full exercise while simultaneously training your nervous system to acclimate to the unusual movement pattern.

The first time you try to do a one-arm negative, you will probably drop like a stone. When starting out, it may help to not even think of it as a negative; just try to keep yourself up and let gravity take care of the rest. The closer you get to a full hang, the harder it becomes to maintain control during the descent. Be prepared to spend a lot of time on this step. You'll need to own every inch of the negative!

GIVE YOURSELF A HAND

On the road to the full one-arm pull-up, it's very helpful to practice self-assisted one-arm pull-ups. This can be done a few different ways.

The first method is what's often known as an "archer" pull-up. For this variant, begin like you're about to do a wide-grip pull-up, but pull your entire body toward one hand while the opposite arm stays straight. This forces your pulling arm to do most of the work, yet allows you to assist yourself as needed.

You can also perform a self-assist by holding the wrist of your pulling arm with the hand of your secondary arm. This is sometimes known as a "one-handed" pull-up. Your primary arm is the only one gripping the bar or ring, but your secondary arm can still assist with pulling. Over time, you can progressively lower your assisting hand down toward your elbow. The farther from your wrist you go, the more work your primary arm will have to do. Eventually, you won't need it at all.

Because the one-arm pull-up is a very intense move, you have to be careful not to overdo it. Not only will beginning your one-arm pull-up training be a shock to your muscles, it will also rock your connective tissue and central nervous system.

One-arm pull-up training can be very stressful on the elbow and shoulder joints in particular. Tendinitis is a bitch, and you've got to respect your body or you will pay the price. As such, I recommend practicing these progressions just one or two days per week for the first few weeks, eventually building to three days per week at most.

I also recommend keeping your volume low. Think of your one-arm pull-up training almost like training for a one-rep max in a heavy barbell lift. You can't do it all the time or you'll burn yourself out.

Due to the lopsided nature of using just one arm to pull yourself, some trunk rotation is unavoidable when performing a one-arm pull-up. Your body will naturally twist as you go up. In the beginning, you should use this to your advantage, and practice turning your hand toward your body as you pull. This will cause your grip to rotate from an overhand to an underhand position as you ascend. When performed on a ring, it will rotate to account for this.

Of all the lessons I've learned during my time training for this remarkable feat, the one lesson I'm reminded of again and again is to respect the journey and be patient. The one-arm pull-up is a show of pound-for-pound prowess unlike any other. Only those who possess the rare combination of patience, strength, and determination have a chance to join the ranks of the elite men and women who've performed a pull-up with just one arm.

Are *you* up for the challenge?

TAKE HOLD OF THE FLAME

BY DANNY KAVADLO

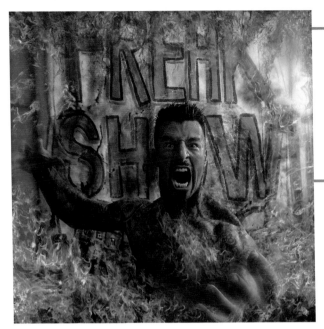

AUTHOR'S INSIGHT:

Any fool can work out when they're motivated. It takes someone special to do it when they're not.

Recently I received an email from a friendly fitness follower. This is what he asked: "Hey, Danny, how do you stay so motivated?" Well thanks for asking! But the truth is: I don't!

That's right. I don't.

There is a fire burning deep within me. It burns within us all. This fire makes me move, helps me survive the night and execute what I must. But this fire is not motivation. There are days when I wake up and I simply don't know what the hell.

- ▶ *How am I going to pay my bills?*
- ▶ *How can I be a better man?*
- ▶ *A better trainer?*
- ▶ *How am I going to feed my son and go on another day?*
- ▶ *And those damn pull-ups.... When can I find the time?*

To evoke California thrash metallers Suicidal Tendencies, "How can I laugh tomorrow when I can't even smile today?"

Sometimes I'm terrified—not motivated at all—but very afraid. Yet somehow, I keep a roof over my head. I work. I cook breakfast. I pay my bills and take my kid to school. And, yes, I do the damn pull-ups. But it has nothing to do with motivation.

The fire within is *dedication*.

If I waited for motivation to strike, I wouldn't do much of anything. My mortgage would go unpaid. My bathroom would be filthy. I'd go days without showering. I certainly wouldn't work out half as much as I want to or need to. It's not that I'm lazy—it's that I'm real and I acknowledge the fact that tasks take effort.

And I'm not sorry to admit, as I type these keys on a rainy Friday morning, that I'm not motivated at all. Instead, I'm accountable. I said I'd write these words on the damn page and I'm doing it, whether I feel like it or not.

The fire within is *discipline*.

We live in the hashtag generation, kids. Everything is *#motivationmonday* or *#flexfriday*. Well, Danny's here to tell you that's a bunch of jive! Do not wait for #motivationmonday! Do not wait for motivation any day!

These slogans are designed to inspire, which of course is a good thing. I'd never deny that. But motivation comes once in a blue moon. It's the great, white whale of lore—an incredible beast to behold—but don't base your life on trying to capture it, or your life may pass you by. Discipline is accessible every day, while motivation comes and goes.

You do the things you choose to do because you care. You do the work every day, whether you're motivated or not, because it's important to you. Be leery of *#inspirational* memes from people you never heard of (or even memes from me.)

The only truth is the truth that takes place in the real world. Virtual reality is not reality and social media is not social. Do not count on others to motivate you. Take care of what you must.

The fire within is *determination*.

Are you "motivated" to brush your teeth? Do you jump up and say, "Hellyeah! It's teeth time!" Or are you determined because it's important for your quality of life? Are you "motivated" to pay your rent, or do you do it because you don't want to live on the street and eat out of a trash can? Are you "motivated" to go to the DMV when you have to renew your license?

You see where I'm going with this, right? In the end, motivation is overrated. It's an illusion. The fire within comes from you, not from any external force. It's your own dedication, discipline and determination. And the flame is strong.

Don't wait for motivation to strike. It may not. Do the thing whether you're motivated or not. Take hold of the flame!

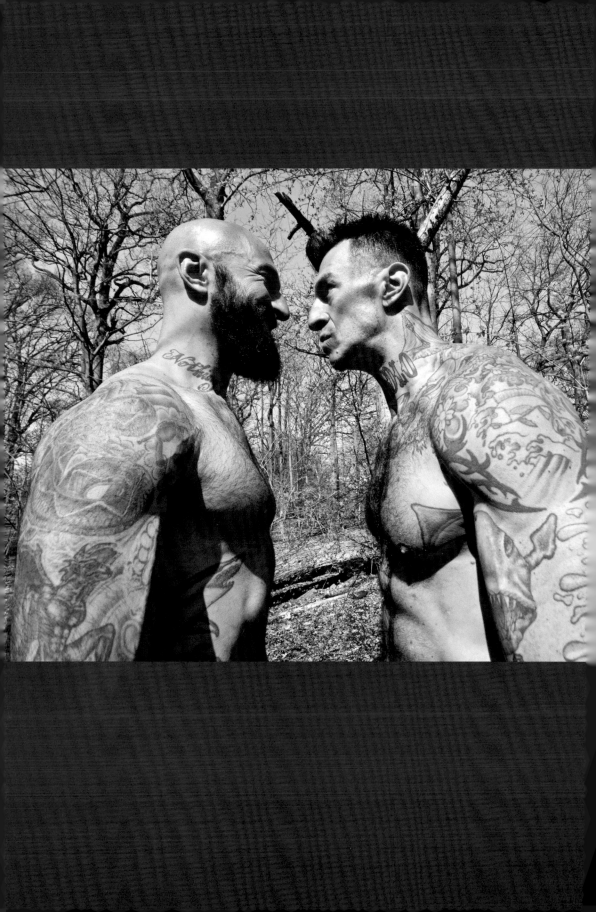

ABOUT THE AUTHORS

Al and Danny Kavadlo are two of the world's leading authorities on calisthenics and personal training. The Kavadlo Brothers have authored several internationally-acclaimed, bestselling books and have been translated into over a dozen languages. They have appeared in numerous publications including The New York Times and Men's Health, and are regular contributors to Bodybuilding.com and TRAIN magazine. As Master Instructors for Dragon Door's acclaimed Progressive Calisthenics Certification, Al and Danny travel the world teaching bodyweight strength training to athletes, professional trainers and fitness enthusiasts from all walks of life. Al is always smiling. Danny is always scowling.

ALSO AVAILABLE FROM THE KAVADLO BROTHERS AND DRAGON DOOR:

Get Strong—The Ultimate 16-Week Transformation Program for Gaining Muscle and Strength—Using the Power of Progressive Calisthenics
By Al Kavadlo & Danny Kavadlo, 2017

Street Workout—A Worldwide Anthology of Urban Calisthenics—How to Sculpt a God-Like Physique Using Nothing but Your Environment
By Al Kavadlo & Danny Kavadlo, 2016

Strength Rules—How to Get Stronger Than Almost Anyone and the Proven Plan to Make it Real
By Danny Kavadlo, 2015

Zen Mind, Strong Body—How to Cultivate Advanced Calisthenics Strength–Using the Power of "Beginner's Mind"
By Al Kavadlo, 2015

Diamond-Cut Abs—How to Engineer the Ultimate Six-Pack—Minimalist Methods for Maximal Results
By Danny Kavadlo, 2014

Stretching Your Boundaries—Flexibility Training for Extreme Calisthenics Strength
By Al Kavadlo, 2014

Everybody Needs Training—Proven Success Secrets for the Professional Fitness Trainer—How to Get More Clients, Make More Money and Change More Lives
By Danny Kavadlo, 2013

Pushing The Limits!—Total Body Strength with No Equipment
By Al Kavadlo, 2013

Raising The Bar—The Definitive Guide to Pull-up Bar Calisthenics
By Al Kavadlo, 2012

INDEX OF EXERCISES

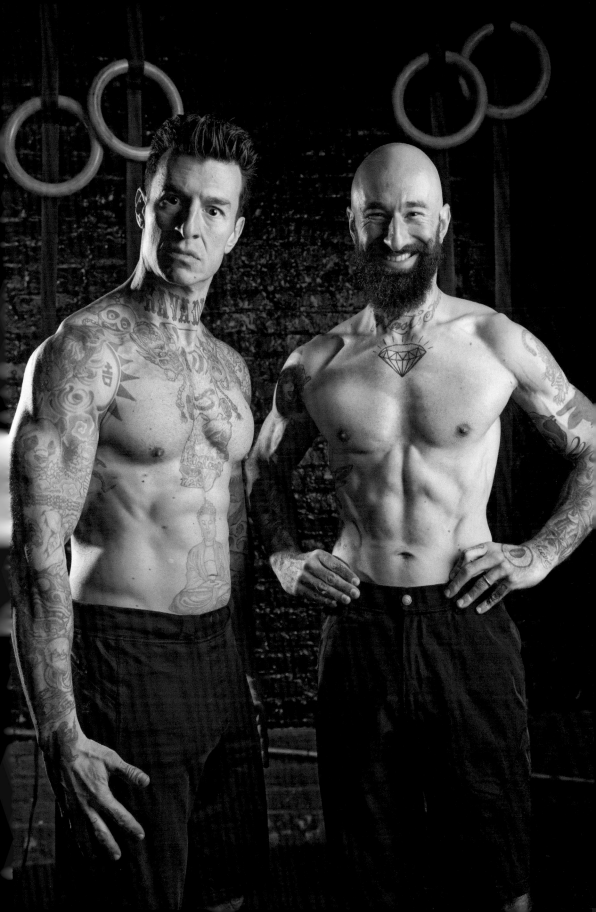

HOW TO BUILD A BETTER BODY *FAST*

Where do you belong on the strength continuum? And where do you want to be?

Too often, we know what we should be doing to gain strength, but we lack direction, a plan, motivation and intelligent guidance to make appreciable gains over the long haul. We have no real goal, no proper focus and therefore underachieve—going nowhere with our strength…

"Get Strong is a phenomenal program. In this book, the Kavadlo Brothers will guide you from the very beginning and help you build a proper foundation. From there, they'll gradually progress you through four phases of strength, giving you the progressions and programing details to take you beyond what you ever thought possible."

—**MARK SISSON**, author of *The Primal Blueprint*

Get Strong is a guidebook for those who are dissatisfied with their current rate of progress—and who want to effect lasting changes, fast…

Your great advantage with the *Get Strong* program is the intelligent realism of its plan. While the Kavadlo brothers have achieved supreme feats of calisthenics strength—like the one-arm pull up, the human flag and the back lever—they have also spent decades helping thousands of clients meet and often exceed their training goals.

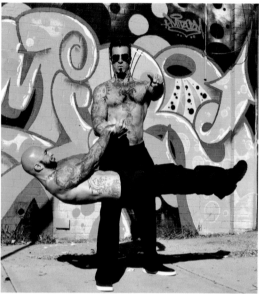

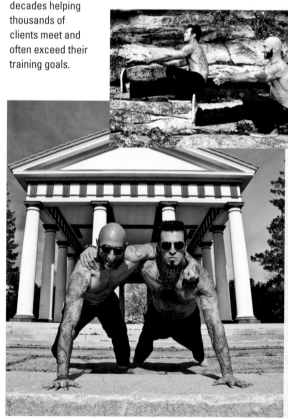

Get Strong
The Ultimate 16-Week Transformation Program For Gaining Muscle and Strength— Using The Power Of Progressive Calisthenics
By Al Kavadlo and Danny Kavadlo

Book #B91 $29.95
eBook #EB91 $9.95
Paperback 218 pages

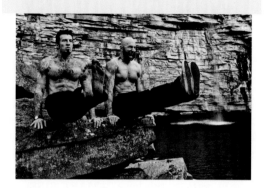

And you can see from their photographs that their choice of exercise regimens has resulted in beyond spectacular physiques. With the Kavadlos' strategies you get strength and looks in one awesome package.

So, you can consider the Kavadlos curators of not only the most effective bodyweight exercises, but also the programming needed to extract the full juice from those chosen drills.

As experienced architects and constructors of strength, the Kavadlos know what it takes to advance from absolute newbie to elite practitioner. The Kavadlos also know how to strip things down to their essentials—to get the most out of the least, the biggest bang for the buck…

You'll discover what key exercises in what exact progressions will give you the best results in the fastest, safest time.

Get Strong guides you through four major phases of strength, using a construction analogy: **Foundation, Brick and Mortar, Concrete and Iron and Forged Steel.** Just follow the master architects' blueprint as drawn—and you cannot fail but to grow a stronger and better-looking body. It's inevitable!

When you graduate from **Phase 3, Concrete and Iron,** you will already possess a beastly level of functional strength—with a body to match.

When you graduate from **Phase 4, Forged From Steel,** you will be at a world elite level for pound-for-pound strength. And the beauty of it all: you can do it!

Once You've Got Strong, Then What?

Once you have completed the **Get Strong** 16-week transformation program, you won't want to stop and rest on your laurels. Because it's all too easy to let entropy take over and to start sliding. Or, per-

The Kavadlos have anticipated your needs beautifully with **Part II, Stay Strong.**

First, Al borrows from his **Ask Al** blog formula and answers most of the questions you are likely to have about the 16-week program. Here's where to go if you're stuck in any manner whatsoever…

Then Doctor Danny delivers the **Dos and Don'ts** of "right conduct" in the quest for bodily fame and fortune. Preach it Danny! Invaluable tips from a man who seen just about everything in the training world, from good to bad to ugly…

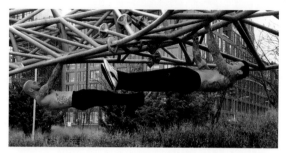

Next, we have a dynamite set of **Supplemental Exercises** you'll want to mix in at some stage. All those Kavadlo favorites that didn't make the cut for one reason or another in the 16-week program: like muscle-ups, flags, dips…

Want variety in your workouts? Sure thing, the Brothers deliver the goods in **Supplemental Workouts**…

Hungry for more variety still? **Partner Exercises** are an awesome way to add fun and challenge to your calisthenics. The Brothers share some of their most iconic moves with you—with some mind-boggling displays of strength.

The Kavadlos are two of the most esteemed and influential article writers on the web. As a great **Bonus Section** in *Get Strong* they have each reworked their five favorite articles to immortalize them in print. Frankly, these ten wisdom-saturated articles are worth the price of admission alone…

24 HOURS A DAY
ORDER NOW
1·800·899·5111
www.dragondoor.com

Order *Get Strong* online:
www.dragondoor.com/b91

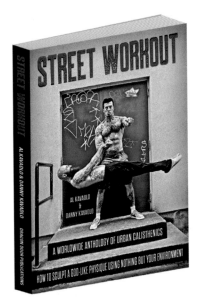

STREET WORKOUT
A WORLDWIDE ANTHOLOGY OF URBAN CALISTHENICS

"Al and Danny Kavadlo—bodyweight coaches extraordinaire—have done it again. Their new book *Street Workout* is an incredibly comprehensive collection of calisthenics concepts, exercises and programs. In addition to their masterful demonstrations of every exercise, the Kavadlo brothers' colorful personalities and motivational talents leap off of every page. If you're serious about bodyweight training, you've gotta get this book!"—**MARK SISSON**, author of *The Primal Blueprint*

Street Workout
A Worldwide Anthology of Urban Calisthenics:
How to Sculpt a God-Like Physique Using Nothing But Your Environment
By Al Kavadlo and Danny Kavadlo

Book #B87 $34.95
eBook #EB87 $19.95
Paperback 6.75 x 9.5
406 pages, 305 photos

"Al and Danny Kavadlo are acknowledged worldwide as masters of urban bodyweight training, so it's no surprise that this book is, without question, the new "bible" of the movement. This work is the greatest manual on progressive calisthenics available on the market today. It's loaded with incredible progressions, stacked with tips and techniques, and overflowing with philosophy and wisdom. The programming sections are beyond extensive. *Street Workout* is THE magnum opus of the two greatest calisthenics coaches on the planet today. All serious athletes and coaches must buy this book!!"—**PAUL "COACH" WADE**, author of *Convict Conditioning*

"I truly LOVE this book—it is utterly sensational and brilliant! Al and Danny Kavadlo have a fun and informative way of explaining and demonstrating the key calisthenics exercises for a fit, healthy and happy life. Their sharp instructional images are joyfully inspirational and always motivate me to bust out some reps on the spot! I truly wish there had been a comprehensive workout guide like this when I first discovered the miracles of bodyweight training."—**MARCUS BONDI**, two time Official Guinness World Record Holder (weighted chin-ups & rope climb)

"Once again, an outstanding addition to our field of fitness from Danny and Al. I am a barbell/kettlebell guy first and foremost, but the Kavadlo brothers have finally convinced me of the pure value of using the body only as load."—**DAN JOHN**, author of *Never Let Go*

"This book brings together the vast knowledge and experience of two guys that definitely embody the whole street workout culture—hardcore, sometimes gritty but always extremely welcoming, with a whole lot of individual style and flare."—**MIKE FITCH**, creator of *Global Bodyweight Training* and The *Animal Flow Workout*

Your Ultimate Guide to Full Body Fitness Without Weights: The Secrets of "Street Workout" Revealed...

How to Release Yourself from the Gym, Restore Your Primal Power and Reclaim Your Inner Beast...

According to the **Kavadlos**, working out should be fun, adventurous, primal and pure. And no training style embodies those elements quite like Street Workout. The outside world becomes your total gym—you roam free to get stronger using simply your own body and the environment at hand...

The great masters of **Street Workout** perform stunning physical feats that can intimidate lesser mortals. But the beauty of the Kavadlos' approach in **Street Workout** is to make even the toughest moves achievable by any enthusiast willing to follow their guidelines. **Street Workout's** multi-faceted, progressive approach leaves nothing to chance— allowing even a raw beginner to transcend his mortal frame and ascend to the giddiest heights of physical supremacy...

Intermediate and advanced calisthenics practitioners will discover a veritable treasure chest of tips, techniques and insider secrets—guaranteed to force-feed their future achievements in the realm of bodyweight mastery.

Pushing, pulling and squatting your own bodyweight along with forward flexion and back bridging represent the basics of getting brutally strong, solid and unbreakable. By utilizing basic principles of progression such as the manipulation of leverage, adding or removing points of contact and/or increasing the range of motion, you can continue to get stronger without ever having to pick up a weight—and have a helluva good time while you're at it!

Street Workout proves it so—with its mix of inspirational photography, exact detail on what to do when—and its step-by-step blueprints for off-the-charts, eye-popping physical excellence.

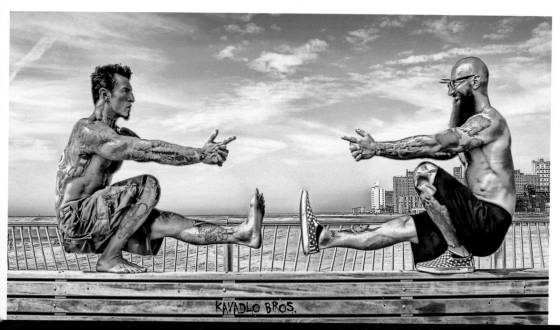

KAVADLO BROS.

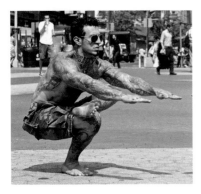
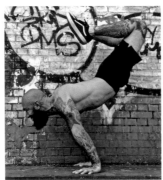
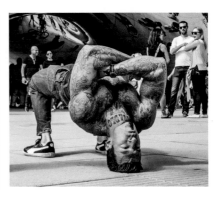

Street Workout fires its first barrage with a crucial section on the **Foundational Progressions**—future and ongoing physical greatness cannot be achieved without mastery of these five fundamental pillars of fitness…

You will immediately appreciate the nobility, virtue and integrity of these movement patterns. Absorb the wisdom of this first section and you have absorbed the very heart and soul of the Street Workout ethos…

CHAPTER 4 awards you the foundational progressions for the **Push**—in all its glory. Discover 30 different progressive drills from the Plank to the Claw Push-Up, to the One-Arm Push-Up to the Hindu Press, to the Ultimate Headstand Press to the Bench Dip to the Korean Dip…

Master all of these 30 moves and you can already tag yourself as a Monster :)

CHAPTER 5 awards you the foundational progressions for the **Pull**—and we're all here for the Pull-Up right? Discover 26 different progressive drills from the Bent-Knee Aussie to the Flex Hang, to the Commando Pull-Up, to the L Pull-Up, to the One-Arm Pull Up…

Look, there is no substitute in strength training for the pull-up—all the more so in our hunched-over world of addiction to devices… And mastery of Chapter 5 earns you the Maestro tag for sure…

CHAPTER 6 awards you the foundational progressions for the Squat—the

ultimate movement needed to build jack hammer legs. Discover 28 different progressive drills from the Bench-Assisted Squat, to the Prisoner Squat, to the Archer Squat, to the Drinking Bird, to the Pole-Assisted Pistol to the Dragon Pistol, to the Advanced Shrimp to the Hawaiian Squat…

Let's face it, you are not a real man or woman without a powerful pair of posts—you are more of a liability to the species… Master this section and you get to represent the species with the Superman or Superwoman tag…

CHAPTER 7 awards you the foundational progressions for the **Flex**—meaning "full body forward flexion". Discover 19 different progressive drills from the Lying Knee Tuck, to the L-Sit, to the Dragon Flag, to the Hanging Leg Raise, to the Rollover, to the Meathook…

Master this section and your etched abs and ripped upper-body musculature will earn you the Mister or Madam Magnificent tag… :)

CHAPTER 8 awards you the foundational progressions for the **Bridge**. Discover 15 different progressive drills from the Hip Bridge, to the Candlestick Straight Bridge, to the One Leg Back Bridge, to the Stand-to-Stand Bridge…

Bridging is an invaluable yet often overlooked component of full body fitness. Bridge work will have a dramatic impact on your power, balance and flexibility—and give you a back that would make a wild tiger proud…

Master this section—along with the previous four—and you can consider your Manhood or Womanhood beyond serious challenge…

So—thanks to mastering the five foundational keys of full body fitness—you can now count yourself as more magnificently in shape than 99% of the human race. But Street Workout encourages you to not stop there, not rest on your laurels…

If you've got this far, then why not shoot for the stars—and enter the immortal ranks of the top 1% of the planet's physical specimens? You can do it! As **Al Kavadlo** and **Danny Kavadlo** themselves bear witness—in photo after photo after photo…

Time to introduce the **SKILLS & "TRICKS"** section of *Street Workout*…

Mastering the exercise progressions in this section will propel you to new heights, to the land where the giants of *Street Workout* strut their splendid stuff. And make no mistake, only the bold of heart, the iron-willed and the profoundly persistent will be godlike enough to make it all the way… If you have those qualities, then nothing should stop you—because the complete blueprint for mastery is laid out for you…

If you are one of those folk looking for cheap hacks so you can pretend your way to greater strength, then this section of *Street Workout* is not for you… However, if you are made of sterner stuff, then read on…

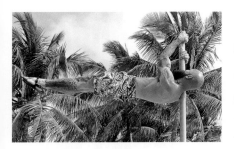
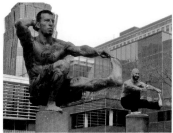
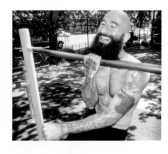

Exercises like the muscle-up, the handstand or the human flag demand the perfect mix of technical skill, hard training and thousands of progressive reps to attain. The Floor Holds, Bar Moves and Human Flag categories within this section contain the instructions you need to make it to the summit. The rest is up to you…

CHAPTER 9 awards you the progressions for Floor Holds. Discover 34 different progressive drills from the Frog Stand, to the One Arm/One Leg Crow, to the Ultimate Headstand, to the Straddle Handstand, to the One Arm handstand, to the One Arm Elbow Lever, to the Scorpion Planche…

The final category to achieve here is the Planche which represents calisthenics strength, precision, skill and fortitude in the most advanced forms. Have at it and let us know how you do!

CHAPTER 10 awards you the progressions for Bar Moves. Discover 20 different progressive drills from the Muscle-Up, to Skinning the Cat, to the Back Lever, to the Front Lever…

Nothing screams *"Street Workout"* like bar moves. Many practitioners of advanced calisthenics were roped in the first time they saw these exercises because they are so spectacular looking. The Kavadlos sure were!

However, these bar moves are not just eye-poppingly cool to look at—they require tremendous strength, skill and perseverance to attain. These gravity-defying feats will suspend you in mid-air and have you feeling like king or queen of the world!

CHAPTER 11 awards you the progressions for the **Human Flag**. Discover 25 different progressive drills from the Side Plank, to the Clutch Flag, to the Support Press, to the Vertical Flag, to the Human Flag Crucifix, to the One Arm Flag, to the Human Flag…

The full press flag has become synonymous with Street Workout. Perform it in public and watch as heads swivel, jaws drop, hearts pound and iPhones leap into action like there's no tomorrow!

Again, though, beyond the amazing visual, there is an ungodly amount of upper body strength needed to perform the numerous types of human flag. Flags will give you—and require—beastly arms, shoulders, an iron chest and a back of sprung steel. The good news is that this chapter lays out the complete blueprint on how to go from Flag-newbie to Human Flag hellraiser…

SECTION IV of *Street Workout* addresses the crucial matter of Programming…

CHAPTER 12 gives you a handy set of **Assessments** so you can see how you stack up against the best in the bodyweight kingdom. Here you can assess your relative calisthenics competency across a broad array of classic street workout exercises. These charts can also serve as a guideline to help you determine when it is appropriate to move on to harder exercises.

CHAPTER 13, Street Workouts, gives you 12 routines to follow or adapt that run from moderate to diabolical in their intensity…

Go from the modest **Start Me Up**, take the **50 Rep Challenge**, say hello to the **Three Amigos,** charge yourself up with **Static Electricity**, split yourself in half with **Up Above** and **Down Below**, bring it and bear it with the Full Frontal, be a sucker for punishment with **Back For More**, magically get the highest possible strength gains with the **Wizard's Cauldron**, scorch your upper body with **Danny's Inferno**, brutalize your horrified posts with **Leg Daze** and finally—for the ultimate of Street Workout warrior challenges—take on the **Destroyer of Worlds!**

CHAPTER 14 gives you 6 **Training Templates** that you can incorporate into your programming. They serve as examples of how you can approach your routines.

A final **BONUS SECTION** brings invaluable additional advice from Al and Danny which pulls the whole Street Workout shebang together, based on questions they've been asked over the years as trainers.

Street Workout
A Worldwide Anthology of Urban Calisthenics: How to Sculpt a God-Like Physique Using Nothing But Your Environment
By Al Kavadlo and Danny Kavadlo

Book #B87 $34.95
eBook #EB87 $19.95
Paperback 6.75 x 9.5
406 pages, 305 photos

How to Get Stronger Than Almost Anyone— And The Proven Plan to Make It Real

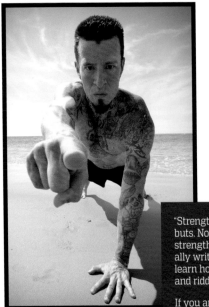

How to Be Tough as Nails— Whatever You Do, Wherever You Go, Whenever You Need it...

Want to get classically strong—in every dimension of your life— gut, heart and mind...?

In other words, do you want to be:

- **More than** just gym-strong?
- **More than** just functionally strong?
- **More than** just sport-specifically strong?
- **More than** just butt-kicker strong?
- And—certainly—**more than** just look-pretty-in-a-bodybuilding-contest strong?

Do you demand—instead—to be:

- Tensile Strong?
- Versatile Strong?
- Pound-for-Pound Strong?
- The Ultimate Physical Dynamo?
- A Mental Powerhouse?
- A Spiritual Force?
- An Emotional Rock?

Then welcome to **Danny's World**... the world of *Strength Rules*— where you can stand tall on a rock-solid foundation of classic strength principles...Arm-in-arm with a world leader in the modern calisthenics movement...

Then... with Danny as your constant guide, grow taller and ever-stronger—in all aspects of your life and being—with a Master Blueprint of progressive calisthenic training where the sky's the limit on your possible progress...

Do Danny's classical **Strength Rules**—and, for sure, you can own the keys to the strength kingdom...

Ignore Danny's classical **Strength Rules**—break them, twist them, lame-ass them, screw with them—then doom yourself to staying stuck in idle as a perpetual strength mediocrity...

The choice is yours!

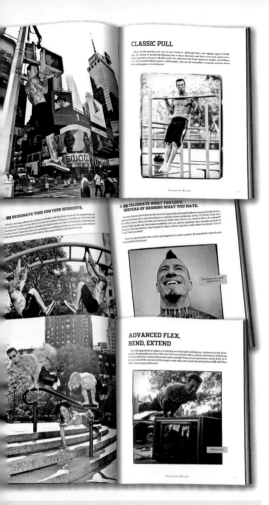

However brilliant most strength books might be, 99% of them have a fatal flaw...

99% of otherwise excellent strength books focus on only one aspect of strength: how to get physically stronger through physical exercise. Health and multi-dimensional well-being is given at best a cursory nod... Nutritional advice is most often a thinly disguised pitch for a supplement line...

If you want a book that gives you the goods on full-body training, full-body health and full-body strength, then there's precious little out there... So, thank God for the advent of *Strength Rules*!

Strength Rules embodies all elements of strength—even how they work into our day-to-day existence, the highs and lows of our being, for better or for worse...

Strength Rules is dedicated to those who are down with the cause. Those who want to work hard to get strong. Who insist they deserve to build their own muscle, release their own endorphins and synthesize *their own* hormones.

Strength Rules has no interest in fly-by-night fitness fads. Classic exercises have stood the test of time for a reason. *Strength Rules* shouts a loud "just say no!" to cumbersome, complicated workout equipment. *Strength Rules* walks a path free from trendy diets, gratuitous chemical concoctions and useless gear...

Almost every strength exercise comes down to the basics. Essentially, Squat, Push and Pull. These three broad, essential movements are the granddaddies of 'em all. Throw in some Flexion, Transverse Bends and Extension, and you've got yourself the tools for a lifetime of full body strength training... That's why the exercises contained in *Strength Rules* are divided into these few, broad categories. Everything else is a variation. There is no reason to overcomplicate it.

The *Strength Rules* mission is to help anybody and everybody get in the best shape of their lives Strength Rules lays out the truth clearly and succinctly, giving you the tools you need to grow stronger and persevere in this mad world—with your head held high and your body lean and powerful.

The exercise portion of *Strength Rules* (titled ACTIONS) is split into three levels: Basic Training (Starting Out), Beast Mode (Classic Strength) and Like A Boss (Advanced Moves). Naturally, not everyone will fall 100% into one of these groups for all exercises in all categories and that's fine. In fact, it's likely that even the same individual's level will vary from move to move. That's cool; we all progress at different rates. Respect and acknowledge it. Trust your instincts.

Speaking of instincts, we are wired with them for a reason. If our instincts are wrong then that's millions of years of evolution lying to us. A large part of *Strength Rules* embraces empowerment, faith in oneself and emotional awareness. Danny believes that being honest with yourself, physically, mentally and spiritually is a magnificent (and necessary) component of true, overall strength. Yes, sometimes the truth hurts, but it must be embraced if we are ever to be fit and free. We all have the power within ourselves. Use it.

Strength Rules cries out to all body types, age groups, backgrounds and disciplines. It talks to the beginning student. It calls on the advanced practitioner, looking for new challenges. It speaks to the calisthenics enthusiast and all the hard-working personal trainers... *Strength Rules* is for *everyone* who wants to get strong—and then some...

Strength Rules by **Danny Kavadlo** is so good you can't ignore it. s minimalistic. It's low tech. It's simple. It's right.

avadlo's work always has me nodding along with a lot of 'yeses' d 'good points.'

his book is about true strength. The old kind of strength where eroes were people, like Beowulf and Ulysses, who protected the mmunity first. This book is about empowering yourself and hers...without stepping on their heads to get to the top.

avadlo quotes one of my heroes, St. Francis of Assisi: 'Start by ing what's necessary; then do what's possible and suddenly you e doing the impossible.' True strength, becoming the best you n be, starts with what one needs to do rather than what one ants to do.

e often ignore calisthenics because of one issue: they are really rd to do. Stop ignoring them. Stop ignoring common sense in trition and supplements. Stop ignoring **Danny Kavadlo**. Again, rength Rules is so good, you can't ignore it."
AN JOHN, author of *Never Let Go*

---

an't say enough good things about **Danny Kavadlo**. I just love s entire approach, mindset and overall vibe. And *Strength Rules* s to be one of the coolest, most badass fitness books I have ever en."—JASON FERRUGGIA

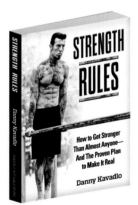

Strength Rules
How to Get Stronger Than Almost Anyone— And The Proven Plan to Make It Real
By Danny Kavadlo

Book #B84 $39.99
eBook #EB84 $9.99
Paperback 8.5 x 11
264 pages, 305 photos

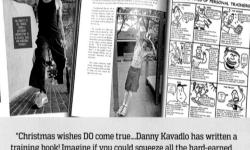
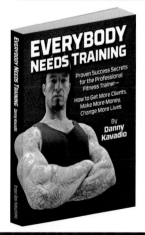

C-MASS

How To Maximize Muscle Growth Using Bodyweight-Only

I s it really possible to add significant extra muscle-bulk to your frame using bodyweight exercise only? The answer, according to calisthenics guru and bestselling *Convict Conditioning* author Paul Wade, is a resounding Yes. Legendary strongmen and savvy modern bodyweight bodybuilders both, have added stacks of righteous beef to their physiques—using just the secrets Paul Wade reveals in this bible-like guide to getting as strong AND as big as you could possibly want, using nothing but your own body.

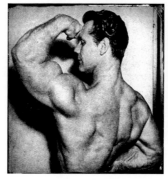
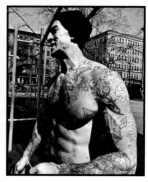

Paul Wade's trenchant, visceral style blazes with hard-won body culture insight, tactics, strategies and tips for the ultimate blueprint for getting huge naturally without free weights, machine supplements or—God forbid—steroids. With *C-Mass*, Paul Wade further cements his position as the preeminent modern authority on how to build extraordinary power and strength with bodyweight exercise only.

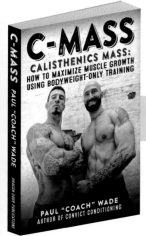

⬇ Get All of This When You Invest in Paul Wade's *C-Mass* Today: ⬇

C-MASS

Calisthenics Mass: How To Maximize Muscle Growth Using Bodyweight-Only Training
By Paul "Coach" Wade

Book #B75 $24.95
eBook #EB75 $9.95
Paperback 8.5 x 11 • 136 pages, 130 photos

1. Bodyweight Muscle? No Problem!

Build *phenomenal* amounts of natural muscle mass and discover how to:

- Add 20-30+ pounds of solid muscle—with perfect proportions
- Reshape your arms with 2-3 inches of gnarly beef
- Triple the size of your pecs and lats
- Thicken and harden your abdominal wall into a classic six-pack
- Throw a thick, healthy vein onto your biceps
- Generate hard, sculpted quads and hamstrin gs that would be the envy of an Olympic sprinter
- Build true "diamond" calves
- Stand head and shoulders above the next 99% of natural bodybuilders in looks, strength and power
- Boost your testosterone naturally to bull-like levels

Understand the radically different advantages you'll get from the two major types of resistance work, *nervous system* training and *muscular system* training.

If you really want to explode your muscle growth—if SIZE is your goal—you should train THIS way...

2. The Ten Commandments of Calisthenics Mass

Truly effective muscular training boils down into THESE Ten Commandments.

COMMANDMENT I: Embrace reps!

Why reps are key when you want to build massive stacks of jacked up muscle.

Understanding the biochemistry of building bigger muscles through reps...

COMMANDMENT II: Work Hard!

Want to turn from a twig into an ok tree? Why working demonically hard and employing brutal physical effort is essential to getting nasty big...

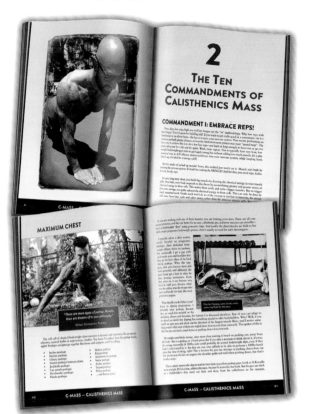

COMMANDMENT VIII: Sleep More!

How is it that prison athletes seem to gain and maintain so much dense muscle, when guys on the outside—who are taking supplements and working out in super-equipped gyms—can rarely gain muscle at all?

Discover the 3 main reasons why, sleep, the natural alternative to steroids, helps prison athletes grow so big...

COMMANDMENT IX: Train the Mind Along With the Body!

Why your mind is your most powerful supplement...

How 6 major training demons can destroy your bodybuilding dreams—and where to find the antidote...

COMMANDMENT X: Get Strong!

Understanding the relationship between the nervous system and the muscular system—and how to take full advantage of that relationship.

Why, if you wish to gain as much muscle as your genetic potential will allow, just training your *muscles* won't cut it—and what more you need to do...

The secret to mixing and matching for both growth AND strength...

3. "Coach" Wade's Bodypart Tactics

Get the best bodyweight bodybuilding techniques for 11 major body areas.

1. Quadzilla! (...and Quadzookie.)

Why the Gold Standard quad developer is squatting—and why you absolutely need to master the Big Daddy, the *one-legged squat*...

How to perform the Shrimp Squat, a wonderful quad and glute builder, which is comparable to the one-leg squat in terms of body-challenge.

Why you should employ THESE 7 jumping methods to put your quad gains through the roof...

How to perform the hyper-tough, man-making Sissy Squat—favorite of the Iron Guru, Vince Gironda—great bodybuilding ideologist of the Golden Era, and trainer of a young Mr. Schwarzenegger. He wouldn't let anyone perform barbell squats in his gym!

2. Hamstrings: Stand Sideways With Pride

Enter *Lombard's Paradox*: how and why you can successfully brutalize your hammies with calisthenics.

Why bridging is a perfect exercise for strengthening the hamstrings.

How to correctly work your hamstrings a[nd] activate your entire posterior chain.

Why THIS workout of straight bridges an[d] hill sprints could put muscle on a pencil.

How to employ the little-known secret of [the] *bridge curl* to develop awesome strength [and] power in the your hammies.

Why explosive work is essential for fully [de]veloped hamstrings—and the best explos[ive] exercise to make your own...

3. Softball Biceps

THIS is the best biceps exercise in the w[orld] *bar none*. But most bodybuilders never u[se it] to build their biceps! Discover what you [are] missing out on and learn how to do it right...

And then you can make dumbbell curls look like a redheaded stepchild with TH[IS] superior bicep blower-upper...

Another great compound move for the b[iceps] (and forearms) is *rope climbing*. As with [all] bodyweight, this can be performed progr[es]sively. Get the details here on why and h[ow...]

Despite what some trainers may ignoran[tly] tell you, you can also perform bodyweig[ht] biceps *isolation* exercises—such as the classic (but-rarely-seen-in-gyms) *curl-[up].* Pure power! If you can build one, THIS old school piece of kit will give you bice[ps] straight from Hades.

4. Titanic Triceps

Paul Wade has *never* met a gym-trained bodybuilder who understands how the triceps work. Not one. Learn how the tr[iceps] REALLY work. This stuff is gold—pay a[tten]tion. And discover the drills that are go[ing to] CRUCIFY those tris!

4. Farmer Forearms

Paul Wade wrote the definitive mini-m[anual] of calisthenics forearm and grip trainin[g] in *Convict Conditioning 2*. But HERE[is a] reminder on the take-home message th[at] forearms are best built through THESE [exer]cises, and you can build superhuman gr[ip by] utilizing intelligent THESE progressio[ns...]

Why crush-style grippers are a mistake[—and] the better, safer alternative for a hand-[crush]ing grip...

5. It's Not "Abs", It's "Midsection"

As a bodybuilder, your method should [be] to pick a big, tough midsection movem[ent] and work at it hard and progressively t[o] thicken your six-pack. This work shoul[d be] a cornerstone of your training, no diffe[rent] from pullups or squats. It's a requireme[nt.] Which movements to pick? Discover t[he] drills here...

And the single greatest exercise [for] scorching your abs in the most e[ffec]tive manner possible is THIS...

COMMANDMENT III: Use Simple, Compound Exercises!

Why—if you want to get swole—you need to toss out complex, high-skill exercises.

Why *dynamic* exercises are generally far better than *static holds* for massive muscle building.

These are the very best dynamic exercises—for bigger bang for your muscle buck.

How to ratchet up the heat with THIS kick-ass strategy and sprout new muscle at an eye-popping rate.

COMMANDMENT IV: Limit Sets!

What it takes to trigger explosive muscle growth—and why most folk foolishly and wastefully pull their "survival trigger" way too many futile times...

Why you need to void "volume creep" at all costs when size is what you're all about.

COMMANDMENT V: Focus on Progress—and Utilize a Training Journal!

Why so few wannabe athletes ever achieve a good level of strength and muscle—let alone a *great* level—and what it really takes to succeed.

Golden tip: how to take advantage of the *windows of opportunity* your training presents you.

How to transform miniscule, incremental gains into long-range massive outcomes.

Forgot those expensive supplements! Why keeping a training log can be the missing key to success or failure in the muscle-gain biz.

COMMANDMENT VI: You Grow When You Rest. So Rest!

If you *really* wanted to improve on your last workout—add that rep, tighten up your form—how would you want to approach that workout? The answer is right here...

Ignore THIS simple, ancient, muscle-building fact—and be prepared to go on spinning your muscle-building wheels for a VERY long time...

10 secrets to optimizing the magic rest-muscle growth formula...

Why you may never even come close to your full physical potential—but how to change that...

COMMANDMENT VII: Quit Eating "Clean" the Whole Time!

Warning—Politically incorrect statement: Why, if you are trying to pack on more muscle, eating junk now and again is not only okay, it can be positively *anabolic.*

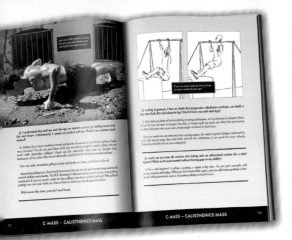

ow to best train your obliques and lateral ...ain...

he simplest and most effective way to train ur transversus...

Maximum Chest

e roll call of classical bodyweight chest ercises is dynamic and impressive. It's ancient, effective, tactical buffet of per-moves. Get the list here...

HE best chest routine is THIS one...

super-sturdy arms and shoulders mean ur pecs barely get a look in when you ..ss, then focus on THESE progressions stead—and your pecs will be burning with a lcome new pain...

ay Al Kavadlo has a lean, athletic physique, his pecs are as thick as a bodybuilder's... .IS could be the ultimate bodyweight drill get thick, imposing pectoral muscles...

d here's the single finest exercise for arging your pec minor—yet hardly anyone figured it out...

y you need to master the art of deep athing, strongman style, to truly develop a ssive chest—and where to find unbeatable ice from proven champions...

Powerful, Healthy Shoulders

die-hard bodybuilders need to know is the deltoids have three heads. Here's they work...

u want to give any of your shoulder ds an enhanced, specialist workout, a t tactic is THIS.

v to make your lateral deltoids scream for cy—and thank you later when you ignore r pleas...

u really want to build your rear delts, S drill should be your number one cise...

ESE kinds of drills can result in shoulder ry, rotator cuff tears, frozen shoulder and nic pain—what to stick with instead...

S is a fantastic deltoid movement which

will swell up those cannonballs fast...

Why old school hand balancing is so great for strength, size and coordination, while surprisingly easy on the shoulders, especially as you get a bit older...

The number one go-to guy in the whole world for hand-balancing is THIS calisthenics master...

8. Ah'll be Back

THIS exercise is the finest lat-widener in the bodybuilding world and should be the absolute mainstay of your back training. This one's a no-brainer—if adding maximum torso beef as fast and efficiently as possible appeals to you...

Are you an advanced bodyweight bodybuilder? Then you may wish to add THIS to your upper-back routine. Why? Well—THIS will blitz your rear delts, scapular muscles and the lower heads of the trapezius. These are the "detail" muscles of the back, so loved by bodybuilders when they grow and thicken, resembling serpents swirling around the shoulder-blades.

Paul Wade demands that all his students begin their personal training with a brutal regime of THIS punishing drill. Why? Find out here...

Real strength monsters can try THIS. But you gotta be real powerful to survive the attempt...

Many bodybuilders think only in terms of "low back" when working the spinal muscles, but this is a mistake: find out why...

How bridging fully works all the deep tissues of the spine and bulletproofs the discs.

The single most effective bridge technique for building massive back muscle...

Why back levers performed THIS way are particularly effective in building huge spinal strength and thickness.

Why inverse hyperextensions are a superb lower-back and spine exercise which requires zero equipment.

9. Calving Season

THIS squat method will make your calves larger, way more supple, more powerful, and your ankles/Achilles' tendon will be bulletproofed like a steel cable...

Whether you are an athlete, a strength trainer or a pure bodyweight bodybuilder, your first mission should be to gradually build to THIS. Until you get there, you don't need to waste time on any specialist calf exercises.

If you DO want to add specific calf exercises to your program, then THESE are a good choice.

The calves are naturally explosive muscles, and explosive bodyweight work is very good for calf-building. So add THESE six explosive drills into your mix...

Methods like THIS are so brutal (and effective) that they can put an inch or more on stubborn calves in just weeks. If you can train like this just once a week for a few months, you better get ready to outgrow your socks...

10. TNT: Total Neck and Traps

Do bodybuilders even need to do neck work? Here's the answer...

The best neck exercises for beginners.

HERE is an elite-level technique for developing the upper trapezius muscles between the neck and shoulders..

THIS is another wonderful exercise for the traps, developing them from all angles.

By the time you can perform two sets of twenty deep, slow reps of THIS move, your traps will look like hardcore cans of beans.

If you want more neck, and filling out your collar is something you want to explore, forget those decapitation machines in the gym, or those headache-inducing head straps. The safest, most natural and most productive techniques for building a bull-nape are THESE.

4. Okay. Now Gimme a Program

If you want to pack on muscle using bodyweight, it's no good training like a gymnast or a martial artist or a dancer or a yoga expert, no matter how impressive those skill-based practitioners might be at performing advanced calisthenics. You need a different mindset. You need to train like a bodybuilder!

Learn the essential C-Mass principles behind programming, so you can master your own programming...

The most important thing to understand about bodybuilding routines...

Simple programs with **minimum** complexity have THESE features

By contrast, programs with **maximum** complexity have THESE features

Why Simple Beats Complex, For THESE 3 Very Important Reasons...

When to Move up the Programming Line

If simpler, more basic routines are always the best, why do advanced bodybuilders tend to follow more complex routines? Programs with different sessions for different bodyparts, with dozens of exercises? Several points to consider...

The best reason is to move up the programming line is THIS

Fundamental Program Templates

- Total Body 1, Total Body 2
- Upper/Lower-Body Split 1, Upper/Lower-Body Split 2
- 3-Way Split 1, 3-Way Split 2
- 4-Way Split 1, 4-Way Split 1

5. Troubleshooting Muscle-Growth: The FAQ

Q. Why bodyweight? Why can't I use weights and machines to build muscle?

Q. I understand that pull-ups and chin-ups are superior exercises for building muscle in the lats and biceps. Unfortunately I cannot yet perform pull-ups. Should I use assistance bands instead?

Q. Looking at gymnasts, I have no doubt that progressive calisthenics methods can build a huge upper body. But what about the legs? Won't it leave me with stick legs?

Q. Coach, can you name the exercises that belong into an abbreviated routine for a total beginner? Which are the most essential without leaving gaps in my ability?

Q. Big" bodyweight exercises such as push-ups and pull-ups may target the larger muscles of the body (pecs, lats, biceps, etc.), but what about the smaller muscles which are still so important to the bodybuilder? Things like forearms, the calves, the neck?

Q. I have been told I need to use a weighted vest on my push-ups and pull-ups if I want to get stronger and gain muscle. Is this true?

Q. Is bodyweight training suitable for women? Do you know of any women who achieved the "Master Steps" laid out in Convict Conditioning?

Q. I am very interested in gaining size—not just muscle mass, but also height. Is it possible that calisthenics can increase my height?

Q. You have said that moving exercises are superior to isometrics when it comes to mass gain. I am interested in getting huge shoulders, but Convict Conditioning gives several static (isometric) exercises early on in the handstand pushup chain. Can you give me any moving exercises I can use instead, to work up to handstand pushups?

Q. *I have heard that the teenage years are the ideal age for building muscle. Is there any point in trying to build muscle after the age of forty?*

Q. *I have had some knee problems in the past; any tips for keeping my knee joints healthy so I can build more leg mass?*

Q. *I'm pretty skinny and I have always had a huge amount of trouble putting on weight—any weight, even fat. Building muscle is virtually impossible for me. What program should I be on?*

Q. *I've read in several bodybuilding magazines that I need to change my exercises frequently in order to "confuse" my muscles into growth. Is that true?*

Q. *I read in several bodybuilding magazines that I need to eat protein every 2-3 hours to have a hope in hell of growing. They also say that I need a huge amount of protein, like two grams per pound of bodyweight. Why don't your Commandments mention the need for protein?*

Q. *I have heard that whey is the "perfect" food for building muscle. Is this true?*

6. The Democratic Alternative…how to get as powerful as possible without gaining a pound

There is a whole bunch of folks who either want (or need) massive strength and power, but without the attendant muscle bulk. Competitive athletes who compete in weight limits are one example; wrestlers, MMA athletes, boxers, etc. Females are another group who, as a rule, want to get stronger when they train, but without adding much (or any) size. Some men desire steely, whip-like power but see the sheer weight of mass as non-functional—many martial artists fall into this category; perhaps Bruce Lee was the archetype.

But bodybuilders should also fall under this banner. All athletes who want to become as huge as possible need to spend some portion of their time focusing on *pure strength*. Without a high (and increasing) level of strength, it's impossible to use enough load to stress your muscles into getting bigger. This is even truer once you get past a certain basic point.

So: You want to build power like a Humvee, with the sleek lines of a classic Porsche? The following Ten Commandments have got you covered. Follow them, and we promise you *cannot* fail, even if you had trouble getting stronger in the past. Your days of weakness are done, my friend…

Enter the "Bullzelle"

There are guys who train for pure mass and want to look like bulls, and guys who only train for athleticism without mass, and are more like gazelles. Al Kavadlo has been described as a "bullzelle"—someone who trains mainly for strength, and has some muscle too, but without looking like a bulked-up bodybuilder. And guess what? It seems like many of the new generation of athletes want to be bullzelles! With Paul Wade's C-Mass program, you'll have what you need to achieve bullzelle looks and functionality should you want it…

COMMANDMENT I: Use low reps while keeping "fresh"!

If you want to generate huge strength without building muscle, here is the precise formula…

COMMANDMENT II: Utilize Hebb's Law—drill movements as often as possible!

How pure strength training works, in a nutshell…

Why frequency—how often you train—is often so radically different for *pure strength* trainers and for bodybuilders…

Training recipe for the perfect bodybuilder—and for the perfect strength trainer…

Why training for pure strength and training to *master a skill* are virtually identical methods.

COMMANDMENT III: Master muscle synergy!

If there is a "trick" to being supremely strong, THIS is it…

As a bodybuilder, are you making this huge mistake? If you want to get super-powerful, unlearn these ideas and employ THIS strategy instead…

Another great way to learn muscular coordination and control is to explore THESE drills…

COMMANDMENT IV: Brace Yourself!

If there is a single tactic that's *guaranteed* to maximize your body-power in short order, it's bracing. *Bracing* is both an art-form and a science. Here's how to do it and why it works so well.

COMMANDMENT V: Learn old-school breath control!

If there is an instant "trick" to increasing your strength, it's *learning the art of the breath*. Learn the details here…

Why inhalation is so important for strength and how to make it work most efficiently while lifting…

How the correctly-employed, controlled, forceful exhalation activates the muscles of the trunk, core and ribcage…

COMMANDMENT VI: Train your tendons!

When the old-time strongmen talked about strength, they rarely talked about muscle power—they typically focused on the integrity of the tendons. THIS is why…

The concept of "supple strength" and how to really train the *tendons* for optimal resilience and steely, real-life strength…

Why focusing on "peak contraction" can be devastating to your long-term strength-health goals…

COMMANDMENT VII: Focus on weak links!

THIS is the essential difference between a mere *bodybuilder* and a *truly powerful human being*…

Why focusing all your attention on the biggest, strongest muscle groups is counter-productive for developing your true strength potential…

Pay extra attention to your weakest areas by including THESE 4 sets of drills as a mandatory part of your monster strength program…

COMMANDMENT VIII: Exploit Neural Facilitation!

The nervous system—like most sophisticated biological systems—possesses different sets of *gears*. Learn how to safely and effectively shift to high gear in a hurry using THESE strategies…

COMMANDMENT IX: Apply Plyometric Patterns to Hack Neural Inhibition

Why it is fatal for a bodyweight master to focus only on tension-generating techniques and what to do instead…

How very fast movements can hugely increase your strength—the light bulb analogy.

The difference between "voluntary" and "involuntary" strength—and how to work on both for greater gains…

COMMANDMENT X: Master the power of the mind!

How to train the mind to make the body achieve incredible levels of strength and ferocity—as if it was tweaking on PCP…

5 fundamental ways to harness mental power and optimize your strength.

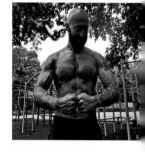

BONUS CHAPTER: 7. Supercharging Your Hormonal Profile

Why you should never, ever, ever take steroids to enhance your strength…

Hormones and muscle growth

Your *hormones* are what build your muscle. All your training is pretty secondary. You can work out hard as possible as often as possible, but if your hormonal levels aren't good, your gains will be close to nil. Learn what it takes to naturally optimize a cascade of powerful strength-generating hormones and to minimize the strength-sappers from sabotaging your gains…

Studies and simple experience have demonstrated that, far from being some esoteric practice, some men have increased their diminished total testosterone levels by *over a thousand percent*! How? Just by following few basic rules.

What rules? Listen up. THIS is the most important bodybuilding advice anyone will ever give you.

The 6 Rules of Testosterone Building

THESE rules are the most powerful and long-lasting, for massive testosterone generation. Follow them if you want to get diesel.

The iron-clad case against steroid use and exogenous testosterone in general.

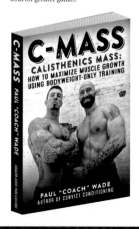

C-MASS

Calisthenics Mass: How Maximize Muscle Grow Using Bodyweight-Only Training
By Paul "Coach" Wade

Book #B75 $24.95
eBook #EB75 $9.95
Paperback 8.5 x 11 • 136 pages, 130

How to Lead, Survive and Dominate Physically—And Reengineer Yourself As "The Complete Athletic Package"…

SUPERHUMAN POWER, MAXIMUM SPEED AND AGILITY, PLUS COMBAT-READY REFLEXES— USING BODYWEIGHT-ONLY METHODS

Explosive Calisthenics is for those who want to be winners and survivors in the game of life—for those who want to be the Complete Package: powerful, explosive, strong, agile, quick and resilient. Traditional martial arts have always understood this necessity of training the complete package—with explosive power at an absolute premium. And resilience is revered: the joints, tendons, muscles, organs and nervous system are ALL conditioned for maximum challenge.

Really great athletes are invariably that way too: agile as all get-go, blinding speed, ungodly bursts of power, superhuman displays of strength, seemingly at will…

The foundation and fundamentals center, first, around the building of power and speed. But *Explosive Calisthenics* does a masterful job of elucidating the skill-practices needed to safely prepare for and master the more ambitious moves.

But *Explosive Calisthenics* doesn't just inspire you with the dream of being the Complete Package. It gives you the complete blueprint, every detail and every progression you could possibly want and need to nail your dream and make it a reality. You, the Complete Package—it's all laid out for you, step by step

"The first physical attribute we lose as we age is our ability to generate power. Close behind is the loss of skilled, coordinated movement. The fix is never to lose these abilities in the first place! Paul Wade's "*Explosive Calisthenics* is the best program for developing power and skilled movement I have seen. Just as with his previous two books, the progressions are masterful with no fancy equipment needed. Do yourself a favor and get this amazing work. This book will be the gold standard for developing bodyweight power, skill, and agility."
—**CHRIS HARDY**, D.O. MPH, CSCS, author, *Strong Medicine*

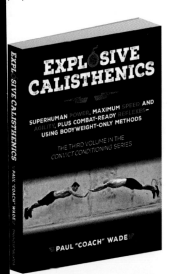

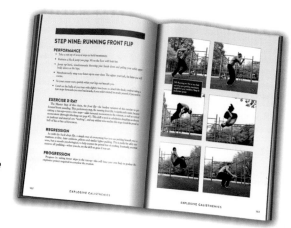

Explosive Calisthenics
Superhuman Power, Maximum Speed and Agility, Plus Combat-Ready Reflexes—Using Bodyweight-Only Methods
By Paul "Coach" Wade

Book #B80 $39.95
eBook #EB80 $19.95
Paperback 8.5 x 11
392 pages, 775 photos

Teach your body to be the lightning-fast, explosive, acrobatic super-hunter your DNA is coded to make you...

With *Explosive Calisthenics*, **Paul Wade** challenges you to separate yourself from the herd of also-ran followers—to become a leader, survivor and winner in the physical game of life. But he doesn't just challenge and inspire you. He gives you the direct means, the secrets, the science, the wisdom, the blueprints, the proven methods and the progressions—that make success inevitable, when you supply your end in consistent, diligent, skillful application.

Now a legendary international bestseller, *Convict Conditioning* can lay claim to be the Great Instigator when it comes to the resurgence of interest in bodyweight exercise mastery.

And—while *Convict Conditioning 2* cemented Wade's position as the preeminent authority on bodyweight exercise—there is no doubt that his magisterial new accomplishment, *Explosive Calisthenics* is going to blow the doors off, all over again.

What makes *Explosive Calisthenics* so exciting—and so profound in its implications?

See, it goes back to the laws of brute survival. It's not "Only the strongest shall survive". No, it's more like: "Only the strongest, quickest, most agile, most powerful and most explosive shall survive." To be a leader and dominator and survivor in the pack, you need to be the complete package...

A vanishing percent of people who workout even attempt to unlock their body's inherent power and speed—choose to be different: reclaim your pride and dignity as a fully-realized human being by fully unleashing your true athletic capacity...

Now—for those who have the balls and the will and the fortitude to take it on—comes the next stage: *Explosive Calisthenics*. The chance not only to be strong and healthy but to ascend to the Complete Package. If you want it, then here it is...

PART I: POWER, SPEED, AGILITY
1: POWER UP! *THE NEED FOR SPEED*

2: EXPLOSIVE TRAINING: *FIVE KEY PRINCIPLES*...P 11

3: HOW TO USE THIS BOOK: *CORE CONCEPTS AND ANSWERS*...P 23

> "*Explosive Calisthenics* is an absolute Treasure Map for anybody looking to tear down their body's athletic limitations. Who doesn't want to be able to kip to their feet from their back like a Bruce Lee? Or make a backflip look easy? Paul makes you want to put down the barbells, learn and practice these step-by-step progressions to mastering the most explosive and impressive bodyweight movements. The best part is? You can become an absolute Beast in under an hour of practice a week. Way to go, Paul! AROO!"
>
> —**Joe Distefano, Spartan Race,** Director of Training & Creator of the **Spartan SGX Certification**

PART II: THE EXPLOSIVE SIX
4: POWER JUMPS: *ADVANCED LEG SPRING*... P 37

— EXPLOSIVE CALISTHENICS —

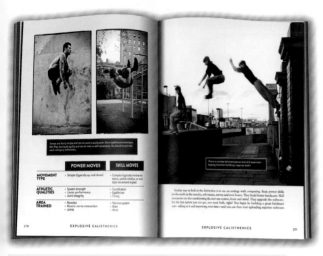

How the clap pushup builds exceptional levels of torso power and quick hands, whilst toughening the arms and shoulders—invaluable for boxers, martial artists and football players.

A killer bridging exercise between clapping in front of the body and clapping behind.

Builds high levels of pure shoulder speed—excellent for all martial artists.

A wicked, wicked move that works the whole body—both anterior and posterior chains.

Get upper-body pushing muscles that are king-fu powerful and robust as a gorilla's…P 98

If God had handed us a "perfect" explosive upper-body exercise, it might be this…P 98

Fast feet and hands go together like biscuits and gravy—here's how to make it happen.

6: THE KIP-UP: *KUNG FU BODY SPEED*…P 109

The mesmerizing Kip-Up is the most explosive way of getting up off your back—and is a surprisingly useful skill to possess. Learn how here…P 109

A fantastic conditioning exercise, which strengthens the midsection, hips and back…P 114

How to generate forward momentum.

Strengthens and conditions the wrists and shoulders for the task of explosively pushing the body up.

Learn how to generate enough lower body power to throw the head, shoulders and upper back off the floor.

Impossible without an explosive waist, super-fast legs and the total-body ability of a panther—which you will OWN when you master step seven…

If there is a more impressive—or explosive—way to power up off the floor, then humans haven't invented it yet…

Master this advanced drill and your total-body speed and agility will start to bust off the charts…P 132

7: THE FRONT FLIP: *LIGHTNING MOVEMENT SKILLS*…P 141

The Front Flip is THE explosive exercise par excellence—it is the "super-drill" for any athlete wanting more speed, agility and power.

Discover how to attain this iconic test of power and agility—requiring your entire body, from toes to neck, to be whip-like explosive…P 141

"Martial arts supremacy is all about explosive power and speed, and you will possess both once you've mastered the hardcore exercises in *Explosive Calisthenics*. Take your solo training to a level you never even imagined with these teeth-gritting, heart-palpating exercises—from a master of the genre."—**Loren W. Christensen**, author of over 50 books, including *Fighting Power: How to Develop Explosive Punches, Kicks, Blocks, And Grappling* and *Speed Training: How to Develop Your Maximum Speed for Martial Arts*

5: POWER PUSHUPS: *STRENGTH BECOMES POWER*…P 73

To round out a basic power training regime, you need to pair jumps with a movement chain which performs a similar job for the upper-body and arms. The best drills for these are power push ups. Here s the 10-step blueprint for becoming an upper-body cyborg…

How to get arms like freaking jackhammers…P 73

How to skyrocket pour power levels, maximize your speed and add slabs of righteous beef to you torso and guns…P 73

How to develop upper-body survival-power—for more effective punching, blocking, throwing and pushing…P 73

How speed-power training trains the nervous system and joints to handle greater loads…P 73

he more power you have in your arms, hest and shoulders, the stronger they ecome. And the stronger they become, e harder you can work them and the igger they get…P 73

ives you an extra edge in strength AND ze…P 73

Vhy the best way is the natural way…P 74

Correct elbow positioning and where to place your hands (crucial)—to spring back with optimal power…P 74

Why cheating with the Earthworm will only rob you—if freakish strength gains are your goal…P 76

How to apply the Myotatic Rebound effect to maximal advantage in your power pushups…P 78

A perfect way to gently condition the shoulders, elbows and wrists for the harder work to come

How to turn your strength into power—and an exceptional way to build your punching force…P 82

A nearly magical preliminary exercise to get better at clap pushups.

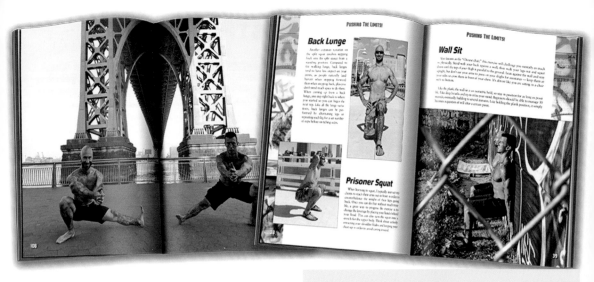

Reader Reviews of Pushing the Limits submitted on DragonDoor.

Time to work smart hard!

"I'm a physical therapist in orthopedics with all the frame wear and tear of a lifter. I use Al's stuff for myself and for patients and always get good outcomes. On my field there are those that make it happen, those that watch it happen, and those that dash in afterwards and ask "Hey, what just happened?" Grab a copy of Al's book. Make it happen."
—GARRETT MCELFRESH, PT, Milwaukee, WI

Al you did it again!

"I'm a doctor that uses functional rehab to get my patients better. This book has helped so much with all the great pics and showing and explaining what and why they are doing these exercises. Also when I get down and show them myself they can see that it is totally achievable! If you are wavering on getting this book, get it! I promise you won't regret it!

From a functional stand point Al, Danny, and Paul are spot on! I've seen and experienced "miracles" from doing these workouts! I have had a bad shoulder, low back, and hyperextended both knees in college football and was told I needed multiple surgeries and was always going to have pain..... WRONG! I am completely pain free and thank these hard working guys for everything they do! I can't wait to see what's next!" —DR. ROB BALZA, Cincinnati, OH

One of the best fitness books I have purchased!

"I recommend this book to anyone who enjoys being active. No matter what sport or training regimen you are currently following, Al's book has something for everyone. Novices and advanced practitioners alike, will find detailed movements that help increase their strength, mobility, and flexibility. Great read with beautiful photography." —LANCE PARVIN, Las Vegas, NV

"I LOVE this freaking Book!!! Every time you put out a new book it becomes my NEW favorite and my inspiration! I love the blend of strength, power, health and overall athleticism in this book! This book covers the BIG picture of training for ALL aspects of human performance.

I will use it with my athletes, with the adults I train, in my own training and absolutely these books will be the books I share with my kids. This stuff reminds me of the old school *Strength & Health Magazine*, I'm fired UP!"—ZACH EVEN-ESH, author of *The Encyclopedia of Underground Strength and Conditioning*

"This is the book I wish I had when I first started working out. Knowing Al's secrets and various progressions would have saved me years of wasted time, frustration and injuries. The variations of The Big Three and progressions Al lays out will keep you busy for years."—JASON FERRUGGIA

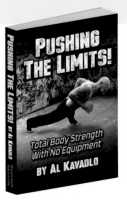

Pushing the Limits!
Total Body Strength With No Equipment
By Al Kavadlo

Book #B69 $39.95
eBook # EB69 $19.95
Paperback 8.5 x 11
224 pages • 240 photos

Sample Spreads From The Interior of *Stretching Your Boundaries*

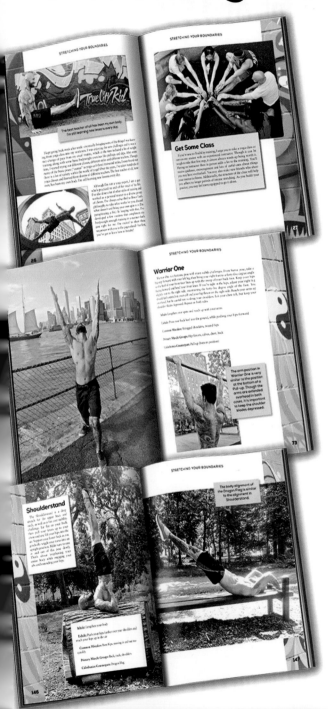

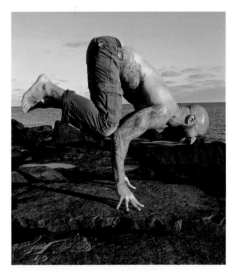

Stretching and Flexibility Secrets To Help Unlock Your Body—Be More Mobile, More Athletic, More Resilient And Far Stronger...

"The ultimate bodyweight mobility manual is here! Al Kavadlo's previous two Dragon Door books, **Raising the Bar** and **Pushing the Limits,** are the most valuable bodyweight strength training manuals in the world. But strength without mobility is meaningless. Al has used his many years of training and coaching to fuse bodyweight disciplines such as yoga, martial arts, rehabilitative therapy and bar athletics into the ultimate calisthenics stretching compendium. **Stretching your Boundaries** belongs on the shelf of any serious athlete—it's bodyweight mobility dynamite!"

—**"COACH" PAUL WADE,** author of *Convict Conditioning*

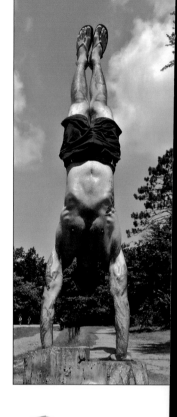

"In this book, Al invites you to take a deeper look at the often overlooked, and sometimes demonized, ancient practice of static stretching. He wrestles with many of the questions, dogmas and flat out lies about stretching that have plagued the fitness practitioner for at least the last decade. And finally he gives you a practical guide to static stretching that will improve your movement, performance, breathing and life. In **Stretching Your Boundaries,** you'll sense Al's deep understanding and love for the human body. Thank you Al, for helping to bring awareness to perhaps the most important aspect of physical education and fitness."

—**ELLIOTT HULSE,** creator of the *Grow Stronger* method

"An absolutely masterful follow up to **Raising The Bar** and **Pushing The Limits,** Stretching Your Boundaries really completes the picture. Both easy to understand and fully applicable, Al's integration of traditional flexibility techniques with his own unique spin makes this a must have. The explanation of how each stretch will benefit your calisthenics practice is brilliant. Not only stunning in its color and design, this book also gives you the true feeling of New York City, both gritty and euphoric, much like Al's personality."

—**MIKE FITCH,** creator of Global Bodyweight Training

"Stretching Your Boundaries is a terrific resource that will unlock your joints so you can build more muscle, strength and athleticism. Al's passion for human performance radiates in this beautifully constructed book. Whether you're stiff as a board, or an elite gymnast, this book outlines the progressions to take your body and performance to a new level."

—**CHAD WATERBURY, M.S.,** author of *Huge in a Hurry*

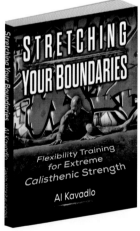

"Al Kavadlo has done it again! He's created yet another incredible resource that I wish I had twenty years ago. Finding great material on flexibility training that actually enhances your strength is like trying to find a needle in a haystack. But look no further, because **Stretching Your Boundaries** is exactly what you need."

—**JASON FERRUGGIA,** Strength Coach

Stretching Your Boundaries

Flexibility Trainin for Extreme Calisthenic Strength
By Al Kavadlo

Book #B73 $39.95
eBook # EB73 $19.
Paperback 8.5 x 11
214 pages • 235 photos

How Do YOU Stack Up Against These 6 Signs of a TRUE Physical Specimen?

According to Paul Wade's Convict Conditioning you earn the right to call yourself a 'true physical specimen' if you can perform the following:

1. **AT LEAST** one set of 5 one-arm pushups each side— with the **ELITE** goal of 100 sets each side

2. **AT LEAST** one set of 5 one-leg squats each side— with the **ELITE** goal of 2 sets of 50 each side

3. **AT LEAST** a single one-arm pullup each side— with the **ELITE** goal of 2 sets of 6 each side

4. **AT LEAST** one set of 5 hanging straight leg raises— with the **ELITE** goal of 2 sets of 30

5. **AT LEAST** one stand-to-stand bridge— with the **ELITE** goal of 2 sets of 30

Well, how DO you stack up?

hances are that whatever athletic level you have achieved, there are some serious gaps in your OVERALL strength program. Gaps that stop you short of being able to claim status as a truly accomplished strength athlete.

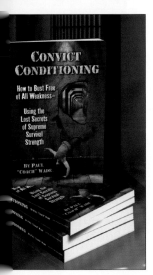

The good news is that—in *Convict Conditioning*—Paul Wade has laid out a brilliant 6-set system of 10 progressions which allows you to master these elite levels.

And you could be starting at almost any age and in almost any condition...

Paul Wade has given you the keys—ALL the keys you'll ever need— that will open door, after door, after door for you in your quest for supreme physical excellence. Yes, it will be the hardest work you'll ever have to do. And yes, 97% of those who pick up *Convict Conditioning*, frankly, won't have the guts and the fortitude to make it. But if you make it even half-way through **Paul's Progressions**, you'll be stronger than almost anyone you encounter. Ever.

Here's just a small taste of what you'll get with *Convict Conditioning*:

Can you meet these 5 benchmarks of the *truly* powerful?... Page 1

The nature and the art of real strength... Page 2

Why mastery of *progressive calisthenics* is the ultimate secret for building maximum raw strength... Page 2

A dozen one-arm handstand pushups without support—anyone? Anyone?... Page 3

How to rank in a powerlifting championship—*without ever training with weights*... Page 4

Calisthenics as a hardcore strength training technology... Page 9

Spartan "300" calisthenics at the Battle of Thermopolylae... Page 10

How to cultivate the perfect body—the Greek and Roman way... Page 10

The difference between "old school" and "new school" calisthenics... Page 15

The role of prisons in preserving the older systems... Page 16

Strength training as a primary survival strategy... Page 16

The 6 basic benefits of bodyweight training... Pages 22–27

Why calisthenics are the *ultimate* in functional training... Page 23

The value of cultivating *self-movement*—rather than *object-movement*... Page 23

The *real* source of strength—it's not your *muscles*... Page 24

One crucial reason why a lot of convicts deliberately avoid weight-training... Page 24

How to progressively strengthen your joints over a lifetime—and even heal old joint injuries... Page 25

Why "authentic" exercises like pullups are so perfect for strength and power development... Page 25

Bodyweight training for quick physique perfection... Page 26

How to normalize and regulate your body fat levels—with bodyweight training only... Page 27

Why weight-training and the psychology of overeating go hand in hand... Page 27

The best approach for rapidly strengthening your whole body is this... Page 30

This is the most important and revolutionary feature of *Convict Conditioning*.... Page 33

A jealously-guarded system for going from puny to powerful— when your life may depend on the speed of your results... Page 33

The 6 "Ultimate" Master Steps—only a handful of athletes in the whole world can correctly perform them all. Can you?... Page 33

How to Forge Armor-Plated Pecs and Steel Triceps... Page 41

Why the pushup is the *ultimate* upper body exercise—and better than the bench press... Page 41

How to effectively bulletproof the vulnerable rotator cuff muscles... Page 42

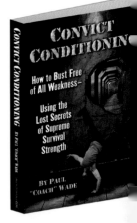

Dragon Door Customer Acclaim for Paul Wade's Convict Conditioning

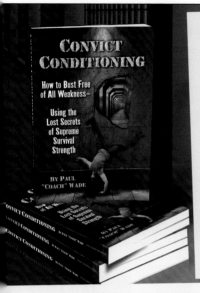

A Strength Training Guide That Will Never Be Duplicated!

"I knew within the first chapter of reading this book that I was in for something special and unique. The last time I felt this same feeling was when reading *Power to the People!* To me this is the Body Weight equivalent to Pavel's masterpiece.

Books like this can never be duplicated. Paul Wade went through a unique set of circumstances of doing time in prison with an 'old time' master of calisthenics. Paul took these lessons from this 70 year old strong man and mastered them over a period of 20 years while 'doing time'. He then taught these methods to countless prisoners and honed his teaching to perfection.

I believe that extreme circumstances like this are what it takes to create a true masterpiece. I know that 'masterpiece' is a strong word, but this is as close as it gets. No other body weight book I have read (and I have a huge fitness library)...comes close to this as far as gaining incredible strength from body weight exercise.

Just like Power to the People, I am sure I will read this over and over again...mastering the principles that Paul Wade took 20 years to master.

Outstanding Book!"—*Rusty Moore - Fitness Black Book* - Seattle, WA

must for all martial artists

s a dedicated martial artist for more than seven years, this
ok is exactly what I've been looking for.

r a while now I have trained with machines at my local gym to
prove my muscle strength and power and get to the next level in my
ining. I always felt that the modern health club, technology based
ercise jarred with my martial art though, which only required body
vement.

ally this book has come along. At last I can combine perfect body
vement for martial skill with perfect body exercise for ultimate
ength.

fighting arts are based on body movement. This book is a complete
tbook on how to max out your musclepower using only body move-
nt, as different from dumbbells, machines or gadgets. For this rea-
it belongs on the bookshelf of every serious martial artist, male
d female, young and old."—*Gino Cartier* - *Washington DC*

e packed all of my other training books away!

ead CC in one go. I couldn't put it down. I have purchased a lot
odyweight training books in the past, and have always been
tty disappointed. They all seem to just have pictures of different
ercises, and no plan whatsoever on how to implement them and
ogress with them. But not with this one. The information in this
ok is AWESOME! I like to have a clear, logical plan of progression
follow, and that is what this book gives. I have put all of my other
ining books away. CC is the only system I am going to follow. This
now my favorite training book ever!"—*Lyndan* - *Australia*

Brutal Elegance.

"I have been training and reading about training since I first joined the US Navy in the 1960s. I thought I'd seen everything the fitness world had to offer. Sometimes twice. But I was wrong. This book is utterly iconoclastic.

The author breaks down all conceivable body weight exercises into six basic movements, each designed to stimulate different vectors of the muscular system. These six are then elegantly and very intelligently broken into ten progressive techniques. You master one technique, and move on to the next.

The simplicity of this method belies a very powerful and complex training paradigm, reduced into an abstraction that obviously took many years of sweat and toil to develop. Trust me. Nobody else worked this out. This approach is completely unique and fresh.

I have read virtually every calisthenics book printed in America over the last 40 years, and instruction like this can't be found anywhere, in any one of them. *Convict Conditioning* is head and shoulders above them all. In years to come, trainers and coaches will all be talking about 'progressions' and 'progressive calisthenics' and claim they've been doing it all along. But the truth is that Dragon Door bought it to you first. As with kettlebells, they were the trail blazers.

Who should purchase this volume? Everyone who craves fitness and strength should. Even if you don't plan to follow the routines, the book will make you think about your physical prowess, and will give even world class experts food for thought. At the very least if you find yourself on vacation or away on business without your barbells, this book will turn your hotel into a fully equipped gym.

I'd advise any athlete to obtain this work as soon as possible."
—*Bill Oliver* - *Albany, NY, United States*

More Dragon Door Customer Acclaim for Convict Conditioning

Fascinating Reading and Real Strength

"Coach Wade's system is a real eye opener if you've been a lifetime iron junkie. Wanna find out how really strong (or weak) you are? Get this book and begin working through the 10 levels of the 6 power exercises. I was pleasantly surprised by my ability on a few of the exercises...but some are downright humbling. If I were on a desert island with only one book on strength and conditioning this would be it. (Could I staple Pavel's "Naked Warrior" to the back and count them as one???!) Thanks Dragon Door for this innovative new author."—*Jon Schultheis*, RKC (2005) - Keansburg, NJ

Single best strength training book ever!

"I just turned 50 this year and I have tried a little bit of everything over the years: martial arts, swimming, soccer, cycling, free weights, weight machines, even yoga and Pilates. I started using *Convict Conditioning* right after it came out. I started from the beginning, like Coach Wade says, doing mostly step one or two for five out of the six exercises. I work out 3 to 5 times a week, usually for 30 to 45 minutes.

Long story short, my weight went up 14 pounds (I was not trying to gain weight) but my body fat percentage dropped two percent. That translates into approximately 19 pounds of lean muscle gained in two months! I've never gotten this kind of results with anything else I've ever done. Now I have pretty much stopped lifting weights for strength training. Instead, I lift once a week as a test to see how much stronger I'm getting without weight training. There are a lot of great strength training books in the world (most of them published by Dragon Door), but if I had to choose just one, this is the single best strength training book ever. BUY THIS BOOK. FOLLOW THE PLAN. GET AS STRONG AS YOU WANT. "—*Wayne* - Decatur, GA

Best bodyweight training book so far!

"I'm a martial artist and I've been training for years with a combination of weights and bodyweight training and had good results from both (but had the usual injuries from weight training). I prefer the bodyweight stuff though as it trains me to use my whole body as a unit, much more than weights do, and I notice the difference on the mat and in the ring. Since reading this book I have given the weights a break and focused purely on the bodyweight exercise progressions as described by 'Coach' Wade and my strength had increased more than ever before. So far I've built up to 12 strict one-leg squats each leg and 5 uneven pull ups each arm.

I've never achieved this kind of strength before - and this stuff builds solid muscle mass as well. It's very intense training. I am so confident in and happy with the results I'm getting that I've decided to train for a fitness/bodybuilding comp just using his techniques, no weights, just to show for real what kind of a physique these exercises can build. In sum, I cannot recommend 'Coach' Wade's book highly enough - it is by far the best of its kind ever!"—*Mark Robinson* - Australia, currently living in South Korea

A lifetime of lifting...and continued learning.

"I have been working out diligently since 1988 and played sports in high school and college before that. My stint in the Army saw me doing calisthenics, running, conditioning courses, forced marches, etc. There are many levels of strength and fitness. I have been as big as 240 in my powerlifting/strongman days and as low as 185-190 while in the Army. I think I have tried everything under the sun: the high intensity of Arthur Jones and Dr. Ken, the Super Slow of El Darden, and the brutality of Dinosaur Training Brooks Kubic made famous.

This is one of the BEST books I've ever read on real strength training which also covers other just as important aspects of health; like staying injury free, feeling healthy and becoming flexible. It's an excellent book. He tells you the why and the how with his progressive plan. This book is a GOLD MINE and worth 100 times what I paid for it!"
—*Horst* - Woburn, MA

This book sets the standard, ladies and gentlemen

"It's difficult to describe just how much this book means to me. I've been training hard since I was in the RAF nearly ten years ago, and to say this book is a breakthrough is an understatement. How often do you really read something so new, so fresh? This book contains a complete new system of calisthenics drawn from American prison training methods. When I say 'system' I mean it. It's complete (rank beginner to expert), it's comprehensive (all the exercises and photos are here), it's graded (progressions from exercise to exercise are smooth and pre-determined) and it's totally original. Whether you love or hate the author, you have to listen to him. And you will learn something. This book just makes SENSE. In twenty years people will still be buying it."—Andy McMann - Ponty, Wales, GB

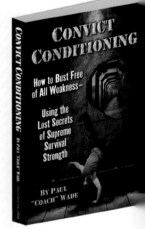

The Experts Give High Praise to Convict Conditioning 2

"Coach Paul Wade has outdone himself. His first book *Convict Conditioning* is to my mind THE BEST book ever written on bodyweight conditioning. Hands down. Now, with the sequel *Convict Conditioning 2*, Coach Wade takes us even deeper into the subtle nuances of training with the ultimate resistance tool: our bodies.

In plain English, but with an amazing understanding of anatomy, physiology, kinesiology and, go figure, psychology, Coach Wade explains very simply how to work the smaller but just as important areas of the body such as the hands and forearms, neck and calves and obliques in serious functional ways.

His minimalist approach to exercise belies the complexity of his system and the deep insight into exactly how the body works and the best way to get from A to Z in the shortest time possible.

I got the best advice on how to strengthen the hard-to-reach extensors of the hand right away from this exercise Master I have ever seen. It's so simple but so completely functional I can't believe no one else has thought of it yet. Just glad he figured it out for me.

Paul teaches us how to strengthen our bodies with the simplest of movements while at the same time balancing our structures in the same way: simple exercises that work the whole body.

And just as simply as he did with his first book. His novel approach to stretching and mobility training is brilliant and fresh as well as his take on recovery and healing from injury. Sprinkled throughout the entire book are too-many-to-count insights and advice from a man who has come to his knowledge the hard way and knows exactly of what he speaks.

This book is, as was his first, an amazing journey into the history of physical culture disguised as a book on calisthenics. But the thing that Coach Wade does better than any before him is his unbelievable progressions on EVERY EXERCISE and stretch! He breaks things down and tells us EXACTLY how to proceed to get to whatever level of strength and development we want. AND gives us the exact metrics we need to know when to go to the next level.

Adding in completely practical and immediately useful insights into nutrition and the mindset necessary to deal not only with training but with life, makes this book a classic that will stand the test of time.

Bravo Coach Wade, Bravo." —**Mark Reifkind, Master RKC,** author of *Mastering the HardStyle Kettlebell Swing*

"The overriding principle of *Convict Conditioning* 2 is 'little equipment-big rewards'. For the athlete in the throwing and fighting arts, the section on Lateral Chain Training, Capturing the Flag, is a unique and perhaps singular approach to training the obliques and the whole family of side muscles. This section stood out to me as ground breaking and well worth the time and energy by anyone to review and attempt to complete. Literally, this is a new approach to lateral chain training that is well beyond sidebends and suitcase deadlifts.

The author's review of passive stretching reflects the experience of many of us in the field. But, his solution might be the reason I am going to recommend this work for everyone: The Trifecta. This section covers what the author calls The Functional Triad and gives a series of simple progressions to three holds that promise to oil your joints. It's yoga for the strength athlete and supports the material in, for example, in Pavel's *Loaded Stretching*.

I didn't expect to like this book, but I come away from it practically insisting that everyone read it. It is a strongman book mixed with yoga mixed with street smarts. I wanted to hate it, but I love it."
—**Dan John,** author of *Don't Let Go* and co-author of *Easy Strength*

"I've been lifting weights for over 50 years and have trained in the martial arts since 1965. I've read voraciously on both subjects, and written dozens of magazine articles and many books on the subjects. This book and Wade's first, *Convict Conditioning*, are by far the most commonsense, information-packed, and result producing I've read. These books will truly change your life.

Paul Wade is a new and powerful voice in the strength and fitness arena, one that is commonsense, inspiring, and in your face. His approach to maximizing your body's potential is not the same old hackneyed material you find in every book and magazine piece that pictures steroid-bloated models screaming as they curl weights. Wade's stuff has been proven effective by hard men who don't tolerate fluff. It will work for you, too—guaranteed.

As an ex-cop, I've gone mano-y-mano with ex-cons that had clearly trained as Paul Wade suggests in his two *Convict Conditioning* books. While these guys didn't look like steroid-fueled bodybuilders (actually, there were a couple who did), all were incredibly lean, hard and powerful. Wade blows many commonly held beliefs about conditioning, strengthening, and eating out of the water and replaces them with result-producing information that won't cost you a dime." —**Loren W. Christensen,** author of *Fighting the Pain Resistant Attacker,* and many other titles

"*Convict Conditioning* is one of the most influential books I ever got my hands on. *Convict Conditioning 2* took my training and outlook on the power of bodyweight training to the 10th degree—from strengthening the smallest muscles in a maximal manner, all the way to using bodyweight training as a means of healing injuries that pile up from over 22 years of aggressive lifting.

I've used both *Convict Conditioning* and *Convict Conditioning 2* on myself and with my athletes. Without either of these books I can easily say that these boys would not be the BEASTS they are today. Without a doubt *Convict Conditioning 2* will blow you away and inspire and educate you to take bodyweight training to a whole NEW level."
—**Zach Even-Esh,** Underground Strength Coach

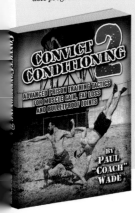

Convict Conditioning 2
Advanced Prison Training Tactics for Muscle Gain, Fat Loss and Bulletproof Joints
By Paul "Coach" Wade

Book #B59 $39.95
Book #EB59 $19.95
Paperback 8.5 x 11
354 pages • 261 photos

Online Praise for Convict Conditioning 2

Best Sequel Since The Godfather 2!

"Hands down the best addition to the material on *Convict Conditioning* that could possibly be put out. I already implemented the neck bridges, calf and hand training to my weekly schedule, and as soon as my handstand pushups and leg raises are fully loaded I'll start the flags. Thank you, Coach!"

— Daniel Runkel, Rio de Janeiro, Brazil

The progressions were again sublime

"Never have I heard such in depth and yet easy to understand description of training and physical culture. A perfect complement to the first book although it has its own style keeping the best attributes of style from the first but developing it to something unique. The progressions were again sublime and designed for people at all levels of ability. The two books together can forge what will closely resemble superhuman strength and an incredible physique and yet the steps to get there are so simple and easy to understand."

—Ryan O., Nottingham, United Kingdom

Well worth the wait

"Another very interesting, and as before, opinionated book by Paul Wade. As I work through the CC1 progressions, I find it's paying off at a steady if unspectacular rate, which suits me just fine. No training injuries worth the name, convincing gains in strength. I expect the same with *CC2* which rounds off CC1 with just the kind of material I was looking for. Wade and Dragon Door deserve to be highly commended for publishing these techniques. A tremendous way to train outside of the gym ecosystem."

—V. R., Bangalore, India

Very Informative

"*Convict Conditioning 2* is more subversive training information in the same style as its original. It's such a great complement to the original, but also solid enough on its own. The information in this book is fantastic-- a great buy! Follow this program, and you will get stronger."

—Chris B., Thunder Bay, Canada

Just as brilliant as its predecessor!

"Just as brilliant as its predecessor! The new exercises add to the Big 6 in a keep-it-simple kind of way. Anyone who will put in the time with both of these masterpieces will be as strong as humanly possible. I especially liked the parts on grip work. To me, that alone was worth the price of the entire book."

—Timothy Stovall / Evansville, Indiana

If you liked CC1, you'll love CC2

"*CC2* picks up where *CC1* left off with great information about the human flag (including a version called the clutch flag, that I can actually do now), neck and forearms. I couldn't be happier with this book."

—Justin B., Atlanta, Georgia

From the almost laughably-simple to realm-of-the-gods

"*Convict Conditioning 2* is a great companion piece to the original Convict Conditioning. It helps to further build up the athlete and does deliver on phenomenal improvement with minimal equipment and space.

The grip work is probably the superstar of the book. Second, maybe, is the attention devoted to the lateral muscles with the development of the clutch- and press-flag.

Convict Conditioning 2 is more of the same - more of the systematic and methodical improvement in exercises that travel smoothly from the almost laughably-simple to realm-of-the-gods. It is a solid addition to any fitness library."

—Robert Aldrich, Chapel Hill, GA

Brilliant

"*Convict Conditioning* books are all the books you need in life. As Bruce Lee used to say, it's not a daily increase but a daily decrease. Same with life. Too many things can lead you down many paths, but to have Simplicity is perfect."

—Brandon Lynch, London, England

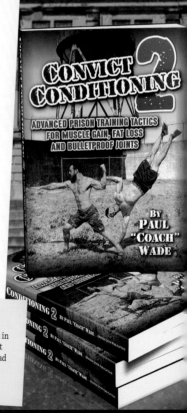

—TABLE OF CONTENTS —

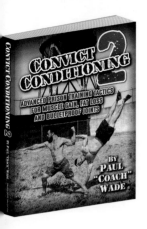

Convict Conditioning 2

Advanced Prison Training Tactics for Muscle Gain, Fat Loss and Bulletproof Joints

By Paul "Coach" Wade

Book #B59 $39.95
Book #EB59 $19.95
Paperback 8.5 x 11
4 pages • 261 photos

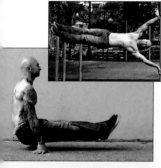

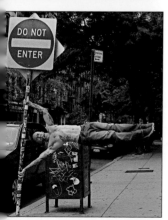

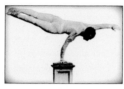

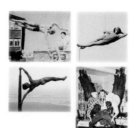

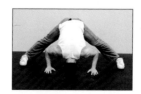

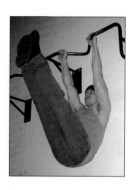

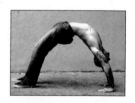

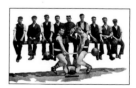

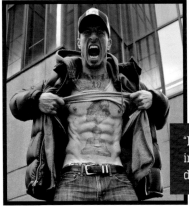

Are You Dissatisfied With Your Abs?

"Diamond-Cut Abs condenses decades of agonizing lessons and insight into the best book on ab-training ever written. Hands down." —**PAUL WADE**, author of *Convict Conditioning*

Are you dissatisfied with your abs? Does it seem a distant dream for you to own a rock-solid center? Can you only hanker in vain for the chiseled magnificence of a Greek statue? Have you given up on owning the tensile functionality and explosive power of a cage-fighter's core?

According to Danny Kavadlo, training your abs is a whole-life endeavor. It's about right eating, right drinking, right rest, right practice, right exercise at the right time, right motivation, right inspiration, right attitude and right lifestyle. If you don't have that righteous set of abs in place, it's because you have failed in one or more of these areas.

With his 25-plus years of rugged research and extreme physical dedication into every dimension of what it takes to earn world-class abs, Danny Kavadlo is a modern-day master of the art. It's all here: over 50 of the best-ever exercises to develop the abs—from beginner to superman level—inspirational photos, no BS straight talk on nutrition and lifestyle factors and clear-cut instructions on what to do, when. Supply the grit, follow the program and you simply cannot fail but to build a monstrous mid-section.

In our culture, Abs are the Measure of a Man. To quit on your abs is to quit on your masculinity—like it or not. *Diamond-Cut Abs* gives you the complete, whole-life program you need to reassert yourself and reestablish your respect as a true physical specimen—with a thunderous six-pack to prove it.

Are You Dissatisfied With Your Abs?

In the Abs Gospel According to Danny, training your abs is a whole-life endeavor. It's about right eating, right drinking, right rest, right practice, right exercise at the right time, right motivation, right inspiration, right attitude and right lifestyle.

So, yes, all of this Rightness gets covered in *Diamond-Cut Abs*. But let's not confuse Right with Rigid. Apprentice in the Danny School of Abs and it's like apprenticing with a world-class Chef—a mix of incredible discipline, inspired creativity and a passionate love-affair with your art.

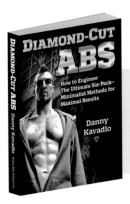

Diamond-Cut Abs
How to Engineer the Ultimate Six-Pack— Minimalist Methods for Maximum Results
By Danny Kavadlo

Book #B77 $39.95
eBook #EB77 $19.95
Paperback 8.5 x 11
230 pages, 305 photos

"Danny has done it again! *Diamond-Cut Abs* is a no-nonsense, results driven approach that delivers all the goods on abs. Nutrition, training and progression are all included, tattoos optional!"— **ROBB WOLF**, author of *The Paleo Solution*

"There are a lot of abs books and products promising a six-pack. What sets Danny's book apart is the realistic and reasonable first section of the book... His insights into nutrition are so simple and sound, there is a moment you wish this book was a stand alone dieting book."—**DAN JOHN**, author of *Never Let Go*

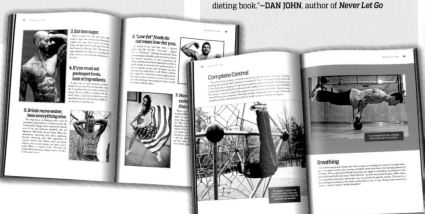

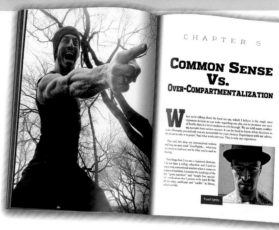

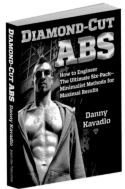
Diamond-Cut Abs
How to Engineer the Ultimate Six-Pack—Minimalist Methods for Maximum Results
By Danny Kavadlo

Book #B77 $39.95
eBook #EB77 $19.95
Paperback 8.5 x 11
230 pages, 305 photos

Order *Diamond-Cut Abs* online:
www.dragondoor.com/b77

1•800•899•5111
www.dragondoor.com

24 HOURS A DAY
ORDER NOW

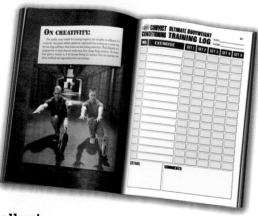
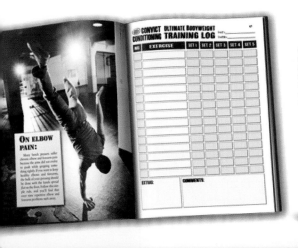
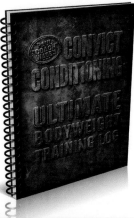

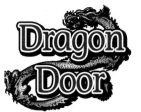

1•800•899•5111 • 24HOURS
FAX YOUR ORDER (866) 280-7619
ORDERING INFORMATION

Telephone Orders For faster service you may place your orders by calling Toll Free 24 hours a day, 7 days a week, 365 days per year. When you call, please have your credit card ready.

Customer Service Questions? Please call us between 9:00am– 11:00pm EST Monday to Friday at 1-800-899-5111. Local and foreign customers call 513-346-4160 for orders and customer service

100% One-Year Risk-Free Guarantee. If you are not completely satisfied with any product—we'll be happy to give you a prompt exchange, credit, or refund, as you wish. Simply return your purchase to us, and please let us know why you were dissatisfied––it will help us to provide better products and services in the future. Shipping and handling fees are non-refundable.

COMPLETE AND MAIL WITH FULL PAYMENT TO: DRAGON DOOR PUBLICATIONS, 5 COUNTY ROAD B EAST, SUITE 3, LITTLE CANADA, MN 55117

Please print clearly
Sold To:
A

Name_____

Street_____

City_____

State _____ Zip _____

Please print clearly
Sold To: (Street address for delivery) B

Name_____

Street _____

City _____

State _____ Zip _____

Email_____

Item #	Qty.	Item Description	Item Price	A or B	Total

WARNING TO FOREIGN CUSTOMERS:

The Customs in your country may or may not tax or otherwise charge you an additional fee for goods you receive. Dragon Door Publications is charging you only for U.S. handling and international shipping. Dragon Door Publications is in no way responsible for any additional fees levied by Customs, the carrier or any other entity.

HANDLING AND SHIPPING CHARGES • NO CODS
Total Amount of Order Add (Excludes kettlebells and kettlebell kits):

$00.00 to 29.99	Add $7.00	$100.00 to 129.99	Add $14.00
$30.00 to 49.99	Add $6.00	$130.00 to 169.99	Add $16.00
$50.00 to 69.99	Add $8.00	$170.00 to 199.99	Add $18.00
$70.00 to 99.99	Add $11.00	$200.00 to 299.99	Add $20.00
		$300.00 and up	Add $24.00

Canada and Mexico add $6.00 to US charges. All other countries, flat rate, double US Charges. See Kettlebell section for Kettlebell Shipping and handling charges.

Total of Goods	
Shipping Charges	
Rush Charges	
Kettlebell Shipping Charges	
OH residents add 6.5%	
sales tax	
MN residents add 6.5% sales	

METHOD OF PAYMENT ___Check ___M.O. ___Mastercard ___Visa ___Discover ___Amex

Account No. (Please indicate all the numbers on your credit card)   EXPIRATION DATE

☐☐☐☐ ☐☐☐☐ ☐☐☐☐ ☐☐☐☐   ☐☐/☐☐

Day Phone: _____

Signature: _____ Date: _____

NOTE: We ship best method available for your delivery address. Foreign orders are sent by air. Credit card or International M.O. only. **For RUSH processing** of your order, add an additional $10.00 per address. Available on money order & charge card orders only.

Errors and omissions excepted. Prices subject to change without notice.

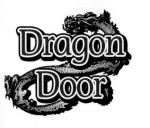

1•800•899•5111 • 24HOURS
FAX YOUR ORDER (866) 280-7619
ORDERING INFORMATION

Telephone Orders For faster service you may place your orders by calling Toll Free 24 hours a day, 7 days a week, 365 days per year. When you call, please have your credit card ready.

Customer Service Questions? Please call us between 9:00am– 11:00pm EST Monday to Friday at 1-800-899-5111. Local and foreign customers call 513-346-4160 for orders and customer service

100% One-Year Risk-Free Guarantee. If you are not completely satisfied with any product—we'll be happy to give you a prompt exchange, credit, or refund, as you wish. Simply return your purchase to us, and please let us know why you were dissatisfied--it will help us to provide better products and services in the future. Shipping and handling fees are non-refundable.

COMPLETE AND MAIL WITH FULL PAYMENT TO: DRAGON DOOR PUBLICATIONS, 5 COUNTY ROAD B EAST, SUITE 3, LITTLE CANADA, MN 55117

Please print clearly

Sold To:

  A

Name_____

Street_____

City_____

State _____ Zip _____

Please print clearly

Sold To: (Street address for delivery) **B**

Name_____

Street _____

City _____

State _____ Zip _____

Email_____

WARNING TO FOREIGN CUSTOMERS:

The Customs in your country may or may not tax or otherwise charge you an additional fee for goods you receive. Dragon Door Publications is charging you only for U.S. handling and international shipping. Dragon Door Publications is in no way responsible for any additional fees levied by Customs, the carrier or any other entity.

Item #	Qty.	Item Description	Item Price	A or B	Total

HANDLING AND SHIPPING CHARGES • NO CODS

Total Amount of Order Add (Excludes kettlebells and kettlebell kits):

00.00 to 29.99	Add $7.00	$100.00 to 129.99	Add $14.00
0.00 to 49.99	Add $6.00	$130.00 to 169.99	Add $16.00
0.00 to 69.99	Add $8.00	$170.00 to 199.99	Add $18.00
0.00 to 99.99	Add $11.00	$200.00 to 299.99	Add $20.00
		$300.00 and up	Add $24.00

nada and Mexico add $6.00 to US charges. All other countries, flat rate, double US arges. See Kettlebell section for Kettlebell Shipping and handling charges.

Total of Goods	
Shipping Charges	
Rush Charges	
Kettlebell Shipping Charges	
OH residents add 6.5% sales tax	
MN residents add 6.5% sales	

METHOD OF PAYMENT ___CHECK ___M.O. ___MASTERCARD ___VISA ___DISCOVER ___AMEX

Account No. (Please indicate all the numbers on your credit card)   EXPIRATION DATE

▢▢▢▢ ▢▢▢▢ ▢▢▢▢ ▢▢▢▢   ▢▢/▢▢

ay Phone: _____

ignature: _____ Date: _____

NOTE: We ship best method available for your delivery address. Foreign orders are sent by air. redit card or International M.O. only. **For RUSH processing** of your order, add an additional 10.00 per address. Available on money order & charge card orders only.

rrors and omissions excepted. Prices subject to change without notice.